HOW TO OVERCOME FATIGUE

inner energy

M.F. Graham, M.D.

With a Foreword by
Kenneth H. Cooper, M.D.
Author of THE NEW AEROBICS

A DRAKE PUBLICATION

STERLING PUBLISHING CO., INC. NEW YORK

Published in 1979 by
by Sterling Publishing Co., Inc.
Two Park Avenue
New York, N.Y. 10016

Library of Congress Cataloging in Publication Data

Graham, Marion Francis, 1919-
Inner energy.

1. Fatigue—Psychological aspects. 2. Fatigue
—Physiological aspects. I. Title.
[DNLM: 1. Fatigue—Prevention and control—
Popular works. 2. Fatigue, Mental—Prevention and
control—Popular works. WM174 G74li]
BF482.G72 616'.047 78-7089
ISBN 0-8473-1802-8

Design by Harold Franklin

Printed in the United States of America

Contents

Appendix

Foreword

As one who has worked with people for over twenty years to help them achieve the optimum in life, I have found that fatigue is a common complaint. It is probably the most common complaint in America today. Even though it is only a state of being, fatigue can be as devastating as any acute or chronic infection. And it is a complex problem. There are many types of fatigue, with different manifestations and different levels of impairment. And as minimal information has been available about management of the problem, the syndrome has plagued both physician and patient for years.

Now Dr. Graham, calling upon his years of medical practice, extensive research, and unusual interest in this field, has analyzed the problem in an erudite, descriptive manner and provided excellent guidelines on the control of fatigue. The beauty of his recommendations is that they can be self-initiated and cost nothing but self-discipline and perseverance.

Dr. Graham, a talented writer and exceptional physician, has a humanism that comes through in his writing. He has taken a difficult subject and with superb descriptions and analogies provided answers for the millions of people suffering from fatigue. If all were to read this book, learn its principles, and apply its recommendations, the results in fuller, more productive and healthier lives would defy the imagination. *Inner Energy: How to Overcome Fatigue* has the potential of doing more for the emotional welfare of its readers than any book on the subject yet published.

Kenneth Cooper, M.D.
Dallas, Texas

PART ONE

The What and Why of Chronic Fatigue

Bill was a forty-five-year-old bank executive who'd been "ladder-climbing" for twenty years, having entered the banking business as a teller the day he got out of college. He owned a nice home, was married to a fine wife, had three great kids, and enjoyed a top-notch reputation in the community. He had made some sound investments, and the only higher rung on his ladder of banking success was to someday become president—provided, that is, one of the other VP's didn't beat him out. The past two years he had noted a nagging fatigue that finally sent him to his doctor with the complaint, "Doc, I'm so tired I even dream of sleeping."

Marilyn was a fifty-five-year-old housewife who, since her children had all flown the coop ten years before, had become increasingly aware of a tiredness that seemed to gnaw at her very bones. "If I hadn't had it so long, I'd think I had the breakbone fever." Her husband traveled most of the time, and she had been so busy raising kids that she had forgotten, it seemed, to give herself a thought, much less a way of life.

Fred was an eighteen-year-old boy who had had things pretty much his own way all of his life. His father died suddenly, and he had to take a job in a filling station to help his mother meet the bills. Not long after he began to work he developed a fatigue problem—so bad, in fact, that he was unable to report for work for as many as two or three days in a row. This had got him fired, and he had sought the help of a physician. "Doc," he said, "it's a major chore to get a foot out of bed in the morning."

As it happened, none of these people had any organic disease. Reams of laboratory tests and X rays brought nothing but normal or negative reports. And this makes them typical of thousands upon thousands of persons who every day besiege their doctors with complaints that go something like this: "Doc, I'm tired all the time." "Doctor, I'm too pooped to pop." "Dead people feel more alive than I do." "Doc, I stay beat." The doctor listens, and questions, then examines, and finally submits the patient to the magic of bloodletting and the wizardry of the roentgen X ray. Eighty percent of the time modern technology spits back nothing but normal findings, and the patient is, essentially, right where he started—tired as hell—only now he's got two or three hundred dollars worth of doctor, laboratory, and X-ray bills to prove it. As a doctor once put it, "I've seen so many tired people that *I'm* tired."

Chronic fatigue is probably the most common complaint heard by today's primary physician—the doctor who sees the patient first. Family doctor, internist, obstetrician and gynecologist, and yes, the pediatrician who sees a high volume of adolescents, know all too well the sad lament sung by a depressed-looking individual sitting on the examining table. It is estimated from various sources that at least half of these individuals have no organic problem whatever. Another third, roughly, may have a minor organic problem that could not possibly account for all the fatigue. And more often than not the complaint is voiced by persons who, by most criteria, are successful people. This led one doctor to the observation: "I believe the world is kept turning by tired people. Maybe that's why they're so tired."

Chronic fatigue may not be an outright killer,* but it is among the most disabling of maladies. As a robber of achievement, a pilferer of potential, it has no peer. It short-changes productivity, dulls ambition, and indeed "makes young men lie upon the bed of the old." More than any other single problem, it leaves the aspirant short of the mark—whether he be mountain climber, bank official, or physician himself.

Physicians generally agree that one of the problems they encounter in dealing with fatigue without organic disease is time to educate the patient. And that is precisely what this book is all about: to help the forever-tired person without a medical problem understand the why of fatigue, and to enable him to use that understanding to solve, at least in some measure, his dilemma.

There is no panacea for chronic fatigue. Let that much be clear. But with a basic understanding of some of the mechanisms involved, much can be done to improve the problem.

Said the patient to the physician after an exhaustive examination: "If I must be tired the rest of my life, I think I am entitled to know why." Said the doctor to the patient: "That you are, my dear lady. That you are. My assistant will call you. I'm too tired."

*Indirectly, however, chronic fatigue probably contributes heavily to suicide, either of the acute or chronic variety. The jaywalker, too tired and tense to make it to the intersection, walks to his death to the tune of several thousand annually. Many a fatal auto accident is triggered by a depressed driver, too tired to cope any longer. Karl Menninger, famous psychiatrist, recounts numerous mechanisms by which depressed, tired persons solve their problems by witting or unwitting self-destruction. (Karl A. Menninger, *Man Against Himself* [New York: Harcourt Brace & World, 1938.])

CHAPTER 1

Fatigue: What Is It?

If you're looking for a capsule definition of chronic fatigue, forget it. The Websterian version, "weariness from bodily or mental exertion," simply doesn't cover the waterfront. So try this one on for size: "Fatigue is a personalistic awareness, an all-pervading sensation, of total energy shortage, wherein the individual feels incapable of meeting the performance demands of any given endeavor with which he is confronted, or does so only with a supreme effort of the will." Complex? You bet. So is the fatigue problem. As a matter of fact, most doctors understand it very poorly, some not much more than the average layman. For fatigue is not only difficult to define, it also defies accurate qualification or quantification. You can't put it under a microscope or weigh it on a pair of scales. That's why it's referred to as a sensation, much in the same manner as pain. It's also an individual thing, that is, it's personalistic; what may be tiring to one individual may not be to another. As you shall see, a lot of input goes into the human brain's returning the computerization known as fatigue. And in the final analysis, that's where fatigue registers—in the brain.

To be sure, you can measure the "fatigue factor" of a steel beam, or of concrete, or of glass, or even of such biologic entities as muscle bundles, nerve fibers, and related physiologic components. But here, as elsewhere in this book, I am talking of the "Doc, I'm always tired" type of fatigue. And that kind defies verbosity, whether with regard to description or to measurement.

Most assuredly, a lot of things can be said about fatigue. But am I really defining fatigue? Let's see.

If a guy says he's weary, pooped, washed out, weak, exhausted, he is saying something—but not with any great precision—about the way he feels. What really happens when such an adjective is used is that a measure of identification is produced between the speaker and the listener. Lives there a man, woman, or child who has never been tired at some time or another and who therefore is unable to identify with such a complaint?

Quantitatively speaking, I suppose such terms as a "little tired," "pretty pooped," or "completely bushed" come as close as any to conveying the degree of fatigue. But unfortunately such terminology does not lend itself to laboratory measurement.

I have a dog who is growing rather old. Time was when he seemed to possess boundless energy, as exemplified by seemingly perpetual motion and an endless desire to chew up whatever was at hand. He was up at the crack of dawn and spent the entire day, I think, chasing shadows, if nothing more. And at night, until I taught him better, he busied himself barking at would-be marauders, imaginary or otherwise. Nowadays, for the most part, he is content to hold down a pad in the shade, and he burns more calories chewing his cud than any other one thing. And he's downright uninterested in what he used to love the most—play. He even looks tired. This is the fatigue of senescence. But it exemplifies many of the symptoms of all types of fatigue: tiredness, lassitude, apathy, indifference, dull affect, mental torpor, difficulty in concentration—in short, the inertia of rest.

In the human being, the foregoing are commonly the earliest signs of fatigue and are for the most part mentally based. As fatigue progresses, as you shall see, patterns of disorganization appear. For example, the couple dancing in a marathon, after two days of ceaseless activity, may be completely unable to walk a straight line. When held out, an arm or a hand trembles. The vision is blurred and hearing is less acute. Muscle weakness becomes overwhelming. In short, with time, the physical signs of fatigue become more and more manifest, and the mental and emotional signs more advanced. Irritability, short-temperedness, depression, hostility, or, at times, manic euphoria—in short, unpredictable emotional display—climb on board the many-carred train that is chronic fatigue the longer restorative measures are denied or withheld.

So when a patient says: "Doc, I stay tired," he is saying a real mouthful. The whole person and the whole of the world in which you live is involved. The mind. The body. The emotions. The past, the present, the future. The ups and the downs and the sideways of life. In fact, the entire gamut of what you are made of and what you have experienced and are experiencing. Your genes, your germs, and your gems. Your rights, your plights, and your fights. Your spouse and your strife. Your muscles and your hustles and your bustles. Come to think of it, "I'm tired" says a whole "bodyful."

CHAPTER 2

Classifications of Fatigue

Acute or Chronic?

The sprinter after the dash; the typist after two or three hours at the keyboard; the cross-country runner after the marathon; the skier after the downhill run; the mountain climber after a day of battling a mountain, all have a fatigue which, though a result of a muscular action differing in duration, shares a common denominator—the energy debt created is rapidly responsive to rest and recuperation. This is the hallmark of acute fatigue. It responds promptly to rest or diversionary activity. Such fatigue may also be the result of mental exertion, as with a prolonged session of reading or study. The emotional component of such fatigue is commonly relatively small in comparison to the physical or mental elements.

On the other hand, chronic fatigue, the type with which this book is primarily concerned, has a clinging, enduring, monotonous character that affects its victim day after day, week after week, year after year. And it is poorly responsive, if at all, to rest or recreation—or if so only on a temporary basis. The emotional component of this type of fatigue is usually very great, out of all proportion to the physical or mental constitutents.

Thus the sprinter, after a few minutes, or the mountain climber after a sound sleep, or the typist after a soda break, are relieved of their fatigue and ready to repeat their performance. Contrariwise, the tired executive, after a night in bed, may feel less like tackling his daily task than when he retired.

Acute fatigue may be superimposed upon chronic states, as you shall see, thus often producing considerable confusion.

Exogenous or Endogenous?

Do the major factors causing fatigue in a given instance arise from within the subject (endogenous) or from without (exogenous)? Workers from cooler climes who pursue the same task in a tropical setting commonly encounter fatigue, an example of an environmental or "from without" fatigue factor. But the football player who, on a sultry afternoon, has not replaced his fluid and salt loss adequately, may feel fatigue long after he has had ample time to rest; his is an endogenous fatigue, although it had an exogenous origin. Other causes of fatigue arising from within are improper nutrition, illness, and nervous states, to name a few.

Briefly, exogenous fatigue is subject to correction mainly through environmental change; endogenous fatigue through change within the individual.

It is obvious that the two are closely intertwined.

Psyche or Soma?

Most students of the subject agree that chronic fatigue never arises solely from physical causes (soma) or solely from mental or emotional ones (psyche). It is an error to try and separate mind from body. It cannot be done. Rather, in any given instance of fatigue, it is a matter of which component, at the time, is the greatest—the psychic or the somatic.

If, for purposes of understanding, you divide fatigue into (1) physical, (2) mental, or (3) emotional, certain facts about fatigue must be kept in mind:*

1. Fatigue is not synonymous with a lack of energy. Rather it is the *sensation* of energy lack that is paramount.
2. Fatigue is not synonymous with decreased productivity, though the latter usually results from fatigue.
3. Fatigue is not synonymous with impairment of performance. There *may* be impaired performance—a sprained ankle in a runner—without fatigue; or fatigue without impaired performance.
4. Fatigue, unlike impairment or injury, is never localized to a given body area. It is an expression of the *entire* individual, a psychic reaction of the whole of the body and mind to a given set of circumstances.
5. Fatigue has a memory. It recalls situations which produced it: Bob had a speech impediment and never felt at ease on the speaker's podium. On every occasion he grew extremely nervous when called upon to speak, and he also grew tired.
6. Fatigue commonly arises out of conflict between the individual and his environment, or out of frustration of the individual in attempting to resolve such a conflict. The individual is said to be poorly aligned with his environment. There is disharmony between the two.
7. Chronic fatigue is ordinarily seen in conjunction with long-term goals and ideas, and long-term self-evaluation of one's adequacy to achieve such goals. The feelings of bodily discomfort attendant upon such malalignment, disharmony, or inadequacy are interpreted as fatigue. In fact, such feelings—the weakness, the limpness, the torpor—*are* fatigue. Without mental perception or awareness, there can be no fatigue.
8. The amount of fatigue commonly parallels a dislike for the task at hand. For example, what overwhelming fatigue commonly besets the teenage boy asked to tun an errand for his father in the family car! Yet how promptly

*Adapted from S.H. Bartley and E. Chute, "Concepts of Fatigue," *Psychology Reviews*, 52 (1945) 169-74. Reprinted with permission.

that fatigue vanishes when he is granted permission to use that same automobile to call on his girlfriend.

From the foregoing, it is apparent that although the ultimate somatic expression of fatigue—inertia—commonly results from fatigue, it is the psychic element which determines such a somatic expression. Thus, the division of fatigue states into physical, mental, or emotional, is an arbitrary one only, and useful only for purposes of dissection and understanding.

Physical Fatigue

Physical fatigue may be of physiologic or pathologic origin. That which follows extensive use of one or more muscles is of *physiologic* origin. This applies whether it is the use of the small muscles of the hand, as in writing, or all the large muscle groups of the body in unison, as in swimming. Certain parameters of physiologic fatigue lend themselves nicely to laboratory measurement, a characteristic not valid for other types of fatigue. Muscle and nerve potentials, reaction time, contractility of muscle, and lactic-acid accumulation are but a few such parameters.

Lesser amounts of physical endeavor lead to weariness without changes that can be measured objectively. If the activity is sufficiently prolonged, there is decreased muscle strength and contractility, along with decreases in the power of concentration and in intellectual performance, as can be demonstrated with psychologic testing. Again, the linkage of physical and psychic components is obvious.

Physical fatigue is of *pathologic* origin when it is due to disease of body organs or systems. In such instances a given amount of muscular activity produces fatigue earlier (in a diseased individual) than in a healthy one.

Mental Fatigue

Pure mental fatigue, without emotional involvement, is a first cousin to boredom, or ennui. It results in feelings of utter relaxation and sleepiness, just the opposite of the irritability and jumpiness seen with nervous fatigue. Thus it relates more closely to physical fatigue. The student who sits down to read a book that is required reading not infrequently finds himself, particularly if the assignment is uninteresting, drifting rapidly into the land of Nod. When a mental task has emotional overtones, such as preparation of one's income-tax return, initial drowsiness may give way to irritability. Repetitious, monotonous tasks requiring little or no thought, as on an assembly line, frequently result in fatigue. Similar work requiring fine eye and finger coordination, as in assembling electronic units, results in fatigue into which the visual and physical components enter to an often unrecognized degree.

Emotional Fatigue

Emotional fatigue is of *psychogenic* origin, just as is mental fatigue. The latter is associated with boredom, monotony, and sleepiness. The former is commonly associated with hurry, worry, and emotional stress; working to capacity in a complex situation; fighting deadlines; struggling against chronic frustration or obstacles with which one cannot come to tangible grips; and attempting to solve problems with ill-defined avenues of solution. Physical and mental fatigue are sleep-producers. Nervous fatigue is a sleep-fighter. The fatigued runner stops and rests. The sleepy puzzle-worker sleeps. But the worried, harried businessperson worries some more.

Most chronically fatigued individuals fall into this group. At the Mayo Clinic 85, percent of one group of patients studied for chronic exhaustion fell into this category. Three hundred cases studied for chronic weakness or fatigue in another series at the Lahey in Boston revealed a nervous state to be at fault in 80 percent of the cases. Thus the odds are heavily weighted that if you complain, "I'm always tired," you fall into one of the following subgroups of emotional or nervous fatigue:

1. Depressions.
   a. Manic-depressive—psychosis
   b. Mild endogenous depression
   c. Involutional
   d. Reactive
2. Neuroses.
   a. Obsessive-compulsive—businessman's syndrome, managerial (from within)
   b. Situational—aggressive-regressive, adaptive (from without)
3. Motivational.
   a. Action-fatigue
   b. Anticipation-fatigue

The Depressions. Fatigue is the handmaiden of depression. The depressed person is almost invariably tired. And unfortunately he often does not realize that depression is at the root of his trouble.

Psychotic depression (manic-depressive psychosis) accounts for only a very small percentage of the depression-fatigue complex. In this group, despon-dency is often confused with true fatigue. These individuals are often "tired of life," so tired in fact, that suicidal tendencies must be carefully watched for. This book does not concern itself with psychotic depression, but it is essential to recognize that it does exist. If you are continually so tired as to be "out of it," incapable of coping with reality on a day-to-day basis, withdrawn, despondent, and dejected ad nauseum, you should not pass yourself off as a mere neurotic. Your problems are, generally speaking, far deeper and of a more serious nature. Psychiatric care is a must.

Out of the psychotic range, but possessing what the famous Dr. Walter Alvarez has termed "poor nervous heredity" or "constitutional inadequacy," are people with "mild *endogenous depressions.*" As shown in Figure 1, the mood swings of the true psychotic are much greater than those of the

Figure 1

MOOD SWINGS IN EMOTIONAL DISORDERS

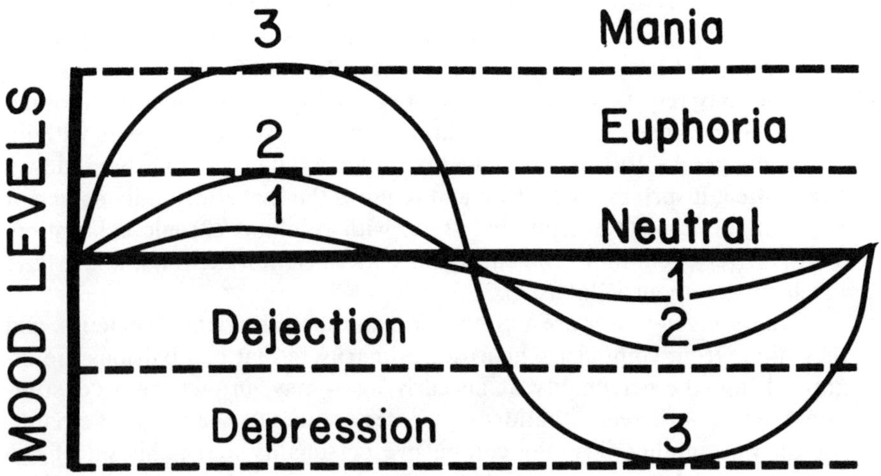

1 = Normal variation from "neutral" mood zone.

2 = Abnormal variation seen in constitutional inadequacy.

3 = Markedly abnormal variation seen in manic-depressive psychosis.

constitutionally inadequate. The mood swings of the latter are nonetheless greater than those of the neurotic. Often there is a fine line between the constitutionally inadequate and the highly neurotic individual. Such disorders tend to occur in families, and affected individuals must often learn to live with the problem, although, as we shall see, much can be done to improve the condition.

Involutional depression is the downswing in mood often accompanying the menopause in the female, and the "womenopause" in the male. It commonly appears in women with the cessation of menstruation, indicating a tapering off of certain endocrine functions. In the male, there is often a loss of libido, a loss of interest in formerly pleasing activities, and a wholesale lessening of activity, both mental and physical. Such depression is physiologic to a degree, inasmuch as it reflects diminished activity of the endocrine system. The accompanying fatigue is often the symptom that takes the patient to the doctor.

Reactive depression is an expected, normal state of dejection or despondency resulting from a despairing turn of events, for example, the loss of a loved one. Normality in an individual so affected is not so much determined by the degree of depression as by its duration, that is how soon and how completely he "bounces back" to his former role in life.

The Neuroses. The company executive who, day after day, week after week, month after month, and year after year, pursues the top rung of the ladder as if his very life depended on it may be suffering from an *obsessive-compulsive neurosis*. Known as the "businessman's syndrome," or "managerial disease," such a neurosis is commonly an all-out effort to over-compensate for early feelings of inadequacy. But burning the candle at both ends can only result, in later years, in a psychologic decompensation, or deflation. Sometimes the balloon of success, inflated over many years with increasingly great effort, bursts suddenly with a resultant nervous breakdown. More often, it springs a slow leak and requires the best effort of its possessor to maintain it in its overinflated state, with resultant chronic exhaustion. This is a very common problem in complex societies like ours, and I have much to say about it later.

Situational neuroses are a dime a dozen in success-oriented societies, and they differ from compulsive neuroses primarily in that compulsions are ingrained into the personality at an early age—may, in fact, be a constitutional defect—whereas situational neuroses are largely the result of circumstance. Put another way, the compulsive personality makes his set of circumstances bad, whereas the situational neurotic is made by his unfavorable environment. For example, the situational neurotic may find himself, not necessarily through compulsion, owning several mortgages and married to a woman who spends their money faster than they can pay the bills. He becomes anxious, sometimes depressed, because of the situation. Fatigue rears its ubiquitous head. The compulsive individual is commonly ambitious, self-centered, pedantic, and perfectionistic, while the victim of a bad situation may be none of these things. He may, in fact, feel quite helpless to attack the problem, whereas the compulsive person attacks so long as he has a breath. Anxiety goes hand-in-glove with neuroses, and is in fact the greatest distinguishing factor between emotionally oriented fatigue and pure mental fatigue. Anxiety always begets tension, and tension always begets fatigue, a cycle so vicious that the most ready solution—a vigorous physical outlet—is often overlooked. Much is said of this later.

Aggression is a hallmark of the compulsive individual, while regression may more commonly mark the situational reactor. Hostility is frequently repressed as the neurotic adapts himself to his obstacle-loaded environment. To the compulsive, it is a world to be conquered at all cost; to the reactor, it is a world to be adapted to in a symbiotic relationship that, at best, means cold and constant warfare.

As we shall see, it is no longer stigmatic, especially in today's complex society, to be labeled "neurotic." Many claim that neurosis is a prerequisite to success. If so, the price is high, but the world is full of persons willing to pay it, as tiring as that may be.

Motivational Fatigue. The gal who awakens in the morning and becomes nauseated at the thought of the work confronting her is suffering from *action-fatigue*. She would like to quit her job and take up something she likes, but circumstances have her hemmed in, forcing her to hold things together. If she has been reasonably successful at her unsavory work, she pursues with a plodding steadiness born of duty. If she has in some measure failed at what she has attempted, whether she likes the work or not, there is an added note of nausea and aversion. If she feels that the task confronting her is too great for her preparation or training, she may be all the more reluctant to undertake it—*anticipation-fatigue.* Motivational-fatigue is not so much the fatigue of "I'm tired" as it is of "I'm tired of." It represents a wish to escape the present or to avoid the future, due to a combination of experience, circumstance, and, sometimes, lack of preparation.

Again, it is impossible to rigidly delineate the different types of emotional fatigue. Depressions and neuroses overlap. Compulsions, situations, and motivation become interlaced. But for descriptive purposes such a classification is helpful. Emotional fatigue is influenced by heredity, environment, and the vagaries of circumstances.

Iatrogenic Fatigue

Don't let the word *iatrogenic* throw you. All it means is "originating with the physician." It is most commonly due to prescribed medications. When you take it in hand to do your own prescribing, as with vitamins, tonics, "rest pills," and other over-the-counter medications, you are commonly unaware that such drugs may have undesirable side-effects, one of which may be fatigue. In today's drug-oriented society, such induced fatigue is quite common, and more is said of it later.

FATIGUE AS THE SUM OF THE PARTS: A UNIFIED CONCEPT

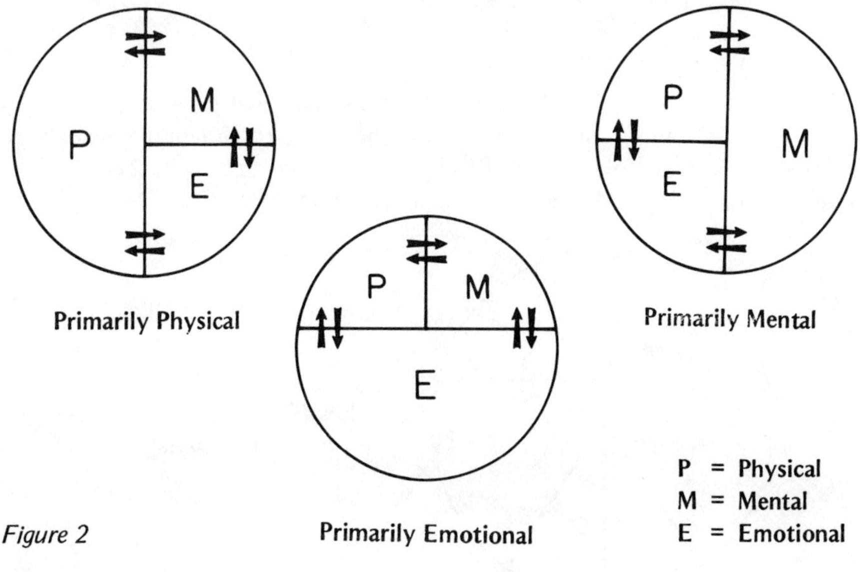

Figure 2

A Unified Concept of Fatigue

To think of any given case of fatigue as being either all physical, all mental, or all emotional, is, as stated previously, an erroneous concept. The businessperson who has sat at a desk all day may be just as bushed as the lumberjack who has felled redwoods for eight hours. And a control-tower worker may be more tired than either when he leaves his tour of duty at a busy airport. Any given case is a conglomerate of all three types, admixed in varying proportions. While the origin of a given case may be primarily physical, primarily mental, or primarily emotional, one component involves the others to varying degrees as shown in Figure 2 on page 21.

The arrows indicate a dynamic interaction occurring among all three factors, so that the degree of involvement of each area in any given situation may vary widely, moreover, from one interval of time to another.

For example, a college track star, the evening prior to an important meet, retires to a quiet corner to study history, a subject in which he has no interest. He soon is fighting sleep, too tired to stay awake. His fatigue state might be represented thusly:

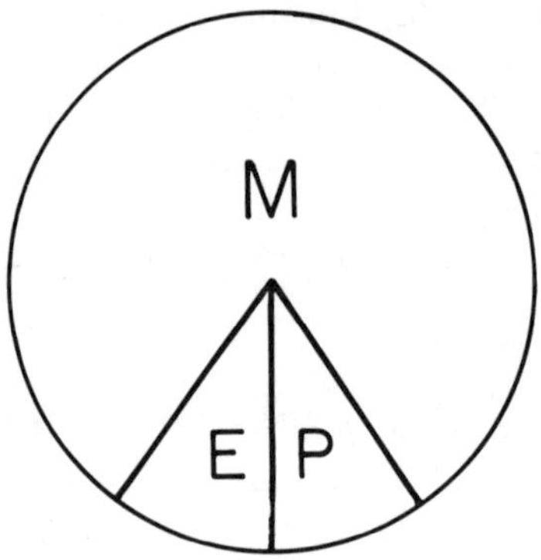

STUDY FATIGUE
(Primarily Mental)

After an hour or two of deep sleep, he awakens and his attention fastens on tomorrow's meet and the competition he faces. He at length gets back to a restless four or five hours of fitful sleep. He feels unduly bushed when he awakens. Now his fatigue state might look like this:

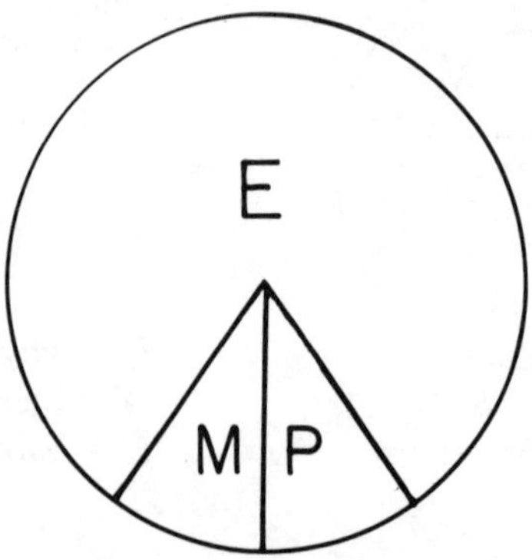

TENSION FATIGUE
(Primarily Emotional)

As meet time approaches, his fatigue sense is replaced by nervous tension and excitement. He runs a good, but hard, race and wins handily. The fatigue he experiences afterward might look like this:

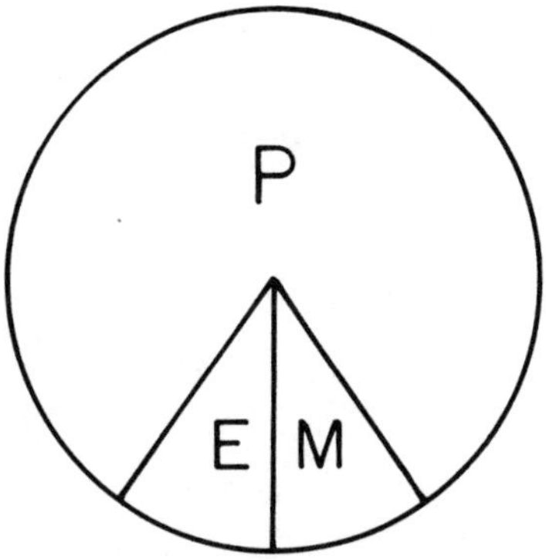

PHYSICAL FATIGUE
(Primarily Physical)

Thus the subjective feeling known as fatigue is the sum of its mental, emotional, and physical components, any one or more of which may at any given time be the major source of the feeling.

Chronic fatigue, the kind which concerns us, is the result of one or more of these components being more or less continuously operative in your life for months or years, without adequate counter measures having been taken at the appropriate time.

CHAPTER 3

Mechanisms of Fatigue

Pathologic Fatigue

Pathologic fatigue is fatigue which results from a physical disease, the kind that can commonly be detected by paying a visit to your doctor. The history, the physical exam, and the laboratory and X ray turn up fatigue caused solely by disease in roughly 20 percent of those who visit a physician complaining of chronic fatigue. Today's diagnostic facilities are quite remarkable. If, after having had a thorough going-over, you are found free of physical disease as a root cause of fatigue, you can generally forget your concern for some hidden abnormality. Many persons—laboring under a phobia of cancer, diabetes, or some other dread disease—are immediately "cured" of their fatigue when they receive their clean bill of health. Others, however, continue to conjure up all sorts of horrible disorders in their minds and merely compound their problem.

While the odds are four to one in your favor of not having an organic cause of your chronic fatigue problem, that one in five chance can represent an abnormality of any organ system of the body—skin, nervous, circulatory, musculoskeletal, endocrine, genitourinary, gastrointestinal, or pulmonary. There is no body system, and hardly any chronic disease of importance, which does not have as a part of its language the symptom of fatigue. And frequently the earliest and only symptom of disease is a nagging feeling of tiredness.

The mechanisms that cause pathologic fatigue are as complicated and as legion as the disease processes themselves. But to provide a bit of insight into some of these mechanisms, let's take a birds-eye look at some of the more common organic causes.

Disease and Fatigue

Obesity. About 20 to 30 percent of American adults are overweight due to too much fat, that is, they are obese. And most, if not all, are tired most of the time. Think of it this way. Joe weighs 180 pounds when his ideal weight is only 150. He is thirty pounds overweight. In a very real sense Joe is carrying a thirty-pound pack on his back—or more accurately around his waist—everywhere he goes. Extra fat contains extra miles of blood vessels to supply the surplus tissue, and extra blood vessels mean extra work for the heart. Moreover, since fatty tissue begets more fat, Joe has to consume extra food just to keep his fat in shape. So fat is a lot like mistletoe on a tree. It partakes of the tree's food supply and offers nothing in return.

In order to meet the extra energy requirements, Joe's heart rate increases, as does his respiratory rate, even at rest. When he is required to do work, breathlessness commonly results. An obese person's respiratory rate exceeds the nonobese individual's by about three times per minute, an extra 4,400 respirations per day. His resting pulse commonly exceeds that of the nonobese by ten beats per minute or about fourteen thousand beats per day. With an increased pulse rate the work of the heart is increased.

The processing of food by the body, known as *metabolism*, requires the expenditure of energy. Thus any intake of calories in excess of what is needed to maintain ideal weight imposes extra work on the metabolic machinery. Digestion, conversion processes, and excretion of end products all require energy. This is one reason why sleepiness commonly follows the intake of a large meal. It is as though the body is bringing its major energy resources into action to manufacture energy supplies from raw materials and to replenish worn-out tissue.

Moreover, high blood pressure and atherosclerosis are two to three times as common in the obese individual as in the nonobese. And these diseases are also causes of fatigue. Diabetes is likewise more likely to develop in the obese, and fatigue is common in the diabetic state.

So fat Joe is overworking his heart and his body machinery if he does nothing more than carry his "pack" around. In addition, like a flatcar in a railroad yard, he is inviting other fatigue producers to climb aboard and add to his load. No wonder fat Joe is usually a tired Joe.

Hypertension. Of the twenty to twenty-five million Americans (about one in ten) with high blood pressure, only half are aware of it. Thus some ten to twelve million Americans are tired because of an unknown elevation in their blood pressure, a readily discernible cause of fatigue. And of the half who are aware of it, only half are under treatment. And of the half under treatment, only half are being treated adequately (following instructions and taking medication properly). That adds up to only one in eight hypertensives who are doing what they should be doing with their disease.

Why is the hypertensive individual tired? The answer is a very complicated one, understood rather poorly by even the experts in the field. Briefly, however, the fatigue which accompanies high blood pressure may be viewed as an effort by the body to lower the pressure, since blood pressure tends to drop with rest.

The mechanics of hypertension involve three major components: (1) vasoconstriction (narrowing) of the small arteries (arterioles) in the body periphery, (2) expansion of the blood volume due to an increased retention of salt in the tissues, (3) a heart that pumps harder than usual to meet the increased loads imposed upon it by (1) and (2).

There are many causes of high blood pressure, but in most instances no explicit cause is demonstrable. That is, a known cause—such as an adrenal tumor, impaired blood supply to a kidney, or disease of a kidney itself—cannot be demonstrated. Such hypertension tends to aggregate in families and is called *essential*, or primary.

The endocrine- and enzyme-system involvement in any case of high blood pressure is extremely complex. When the blood supply to the kidney is interfered with, it secretes enzymes that cause a constriction of the small arterioles. It also causes the adrenal gland to secrete a hormone called *aldosterone*, the effect of which is to retain sodium (present in salt) and in turn to retain water and increase the blood volume. It is as if, by such means, the kidney is attempting to restore a normal flow of blood to its own tissue.

It's a "me-first" attitude on the part of the kidney, and the narrowing of blood vessels which results may account for the feeling of fatigue so common to the hypertensive. The kidney may meet its demands as a result of such measures, but in so doing, it deprives other tissues of blood and thus of oxygen. An oxygen-deprived tissue, whether it be muscle or brain, is a tired tissue. Supporting this concept is the fact that treatment measures, such as vigorous exercise in particular, or drugs which produce vasodilation, tend to counteract fatigue in the mild-to-moderately hypertensive person. More of this later.

The hypertensive person is usually a tired person. So if you're tired and don't know the status of your blood pressure, have it checked. Remember, there's a one in ten chance that this is your problem—a readily detectable and readily treatable one.

Diabetes Mellitus. *Diabetes*, an endocrine disorder affecting some five million Americans, represents an aberration in the metabolism of glucose. Glucose is the sugar present in certain quantities in the blood, and the sugar upon which the body depends in large measure for energy. In diabetes the levels of blood sugar are increased to abnormal levels as a result of inadequate production of insulin by the pancreas, or an inability of the body tissue to utilize insulin in a normal manner. Consequently, levels of fatty materials in the blood increase concomitantly, and the blood becomes sated with certain products of fat metabolism. In essence, when the body is unable to get its needed energy from glucose in the usual manner, it begins to utilize fats, and the result is an accumulation of glucose, fatty materials, and their metabolic by-products in the blood and body tissues. Not only is the body deprived of its customary energy supply, but certain of the other products—the ketone bodies, for example—may even have an anesthetic effect on the individual. Any fatigued individual who is constantly thirsty and urinating large amounts, especially with a strong family history of diabetes (onset before age sixty in a parent, sibling, aunt, or uncle), should be aware of the possibility that he may have the disease and should see his physician.

There are different stages of diabetes, and a negative urine test does not rule out a latent, or preclinical, stage. Blood-sugar determinations are a must in such instances.

Atherosclerosis. *Atherosclerosis*, or hardening of the arteries (arteriosclerosis), is the most common American affliction. It is a disease of affluence with multiple factors entering into its causation, some hereditary and some environmental. No effort is made here to expound upon this very common disease. When, however, atherosclerosis affects a blood vessel, the result is a narrowing of the interior cavity (the lumen) of that vessel by wheylike deposits (atheromata) in its lining, with a subsequent diminution of blood supply to the organ supplied by that artery. If the artery supplies the heart, heart disease may result. If it supplies the kidney, hypertension ensues. If it supplies the brain, a stroke may occur. In a leg muscle, a narrowed artery may give rise to leg pain with muscular endeavor.

Fatigue may result from impaired blood supply (and thus oxygen supply) to almost any tissue, but especially to the brain and kidney. In the latter instance, hypertension may be present, and this process in turn accentuates the fatigue (see above).

Atherosclerosis is an insidious process, often decades in becoming manifest, but there is reason to believe that long before the heart attack, the stroke, or the onset of hypertension, fatigue of otherwise unexplained origin may be a subtle reminder of impaired blood supply to vital organs.

Cancer. Malignant growths of tissue (neoplasms) are composed of populations of parasitic outlaw cells which drain energy for their own reproduction and multiplication from body reserves, crowd out useful cells, and thus decrease vital body functions. The energy requirements for cancerous cells often exceed the requirements of normal cells, so that cancerous growths exist at the expense of normal tissue. Thus fatigue is an invariable symptom of cancer, and wasting and weakness are very common. In addition, loss of appetite commonly supervenes, so that the replenishment of energy supplies is interfered with at the same time that normal tissue is broken down for use in metabolism of cancerous tissue.

The tired patient probably thinks more often of cancer than any other disease, and while this malady claims some 350,000 lives annually, modern detection and treatment is saving thousands more that would have been lost years ago. The main thing to be decried in the conquest of cancer is an ostrichlike attitude. Early detection and treatment give the best shot at a cure.

Arthritic Disease. Rheumatoid arthritis may attack any age group, from young children to older adults. A poorly understood, crippling disease which can affect either the small joints, such as those of the fingers, or the spine, rheumatoid arthritis commonly causes fatigue. The chronic inactivity imposed by the joint deformities and defects augments the fatigue.

Osteoarthritis is a degenerative disease affecting older persons, often relegating them to wheelchair, cane, or rocking chair. The imposed inactivity, again, is a major factor in the fatigue and muscle weakness so commonly accompanying this disorder.

Acute Infections. Acute infections are those running their course in a relatively short time—days or weeks. The common cold, influenza, appendicitis, sore throats, pneumonias, gastrointestinal upsets, and the like are commonly recognized to be accompanied by fatigue and a washed-out feeling. In such instances, the body supplies energy for the growth and reproduction of the invading organisms, a depletion process often accompanied by the release of toxins and other noxious by-products by the organisms themselves. Some infections, such as those causing diarrhea, cause a rapid loss of fluid and nutritive materials and, if accompanied by vomiting, effectually shut off the body's ability to replenish its drained reserves. Thus infections cause fatigue by a variety of mechanisms. Some illnesses, such as influenza, may require weeks after the fever and aching subside before the patient recovers from his washed-out feeling. This period of convalescence represents a phase of recuperation during which noxious by-products of the infection are being removed and drained tissue reserves replenished.

In some instances an acute infection may blend into a chronic disease, and fatigue may remain as a constant complaint for weeks, months, or years after apparent recovery from the acute illness. Examples of this are cases of infectious hepatitis which become chronic, or instances of acute nephritis (kidney inflammation) which merge into Bright's disease (chronic nephritis).

Chronic Infections. Some infectious diseases are characterized by a long, protracted course running into years. Before modern-day drugs became available, tuberculosis was a prime example of this. Leprosy still runs a chronic course. Certain fungus infections of the lung do likewise.

Again, fatigue is a common accompaniment of such ailments, the result of an insidious and inexorable drain on the body resources. Basically, all germs are parasites and extract their own life from the life of the host.

Hypothyroidism. Hypothyroidism and diabetes mellitus are well-known endocrine diseases.* Hypothyroidism, known in its more severe form as *myxedema*, is a deficiency of thyroid function either as a result of inadequate stimulation of the thyroid gland, inadequate function of that gland in manufacturing its hormones, or inadequate function of the hormone thyroxine at the cellular level. While the myxedematous patient presents no problem in diagnosis, the patient with mild deficiencies may go undetected. He is characteristically always tired and sluggish, both physically and mentally. He may have rather puffy eyes, thick (slurred) speech, and doughy skin. His color may be said to be pasty, his hair may be sparse, and his skin dry. His affect is dull and he makes, as a rule, rather poor company. But the borderline cases have been known to go undiagnosed for years, pushing along in an ever-exhausted state out of sheer determination.

Thyroid hormones are essential to the mobilization and combustion of body fuels—sugar and fat. When such fuels are improperly utilized, the

*The endocrine glands are those which secrete vital, regulatory chemicals, called *hormones*, directly into the bloodstream. The best-known of these glands are probably the thyroid gland, the pancreas, and the pituitary.

result is fatigue, just as an automobile with an improperly adjusted carburetor may run tired. Such maladjustment frequently shows up in the thyroid-deficient patient as intolerance to cold, or muscle weakness on exertion.

Today's methods for detecting thyroid deficiency are quite accurate, and there is little reason to miss the diagnosis if it is entertained. The response of such a patient to thyroid medications is nothing short of miraculous.

Immunologic Diseases. There are a host of such ailments, some very involved, but the one with which most persons are in some measure familiar is allergy in one or another of its numerous forms—allergic rhinitis (hay fever), asthma, gastrointestinal allergy, allergic sinusitis, or eczema.

Practically everyone is aware that allergy, depending upon the body system it affects (nose and sinuses, lungs, gastrointestinal tract, skin), may cause stuffy nose, sneezing, tearing, cough, postnasal drip, wheezing, gastrointestinal upset, or a characteristic skin eruption. But most people are unaware of the so-called tension-fatigue syndrome, a collection of symptoms the most notorious of which is a constant feeling of tiredness manifested by uninterest, lackadaisical attitude, and irritability. Such a patient often has a known allergy and, though familiar with his more obvious symptoms, often goes along for years not knowing that his fatigue is just as much a symptom of his allergy as his sneezing. He is not familiar with the fact that the horsehair or the pollen which makes his nose run and causes him to wheeze, or the chocolate which breaks him out, can also render him chronically tired.

But many patients with chronic fatigue, some of whom have been through the mill diagnostically and have been found wanting for organic disease, have unknown or unrecognized allergies, often to food. Foods high on the list for causing such symptoms are chocolate (and cola drinks), milk and milk products, grains, and eggs; but *any* food or combination of foods may be responsible. It is not too difficult for a competent physician to determine such a basis for fatigue, and when seen in conjunction with puffy eyes, drippy nose, and chronic sniffles or cough, allergy should always be suspect.

The precise cause of fatigue in such instances is not known. It may be the result of "immune complexes" that circulate in the blood or affix to body tissues, or possibly a by-product of certain of the chemical mediators released by the allergic reaction. At any rate, the treatment par excellence is removal of the offending agent from diet or environment.

Muscle Diseases. One of the more common causes of chronic fatigue in this group goes by the name of *myasthenia gravis*. Usually the fatigue in such instances is manifest more as a weakness of muscle groups rather than pure tiredness. The defect in this disease is that of deficiency of an enzyme which is necessary for transmission of nerve signals to muscle tissue, or as more recent evidence indicates, myasthenia very likely is an immunologic disease.

Chronic Fatigue and Body Systems

Fatigue may result from an involvement of any of the body systems.

Commonly disease involves two, several, or all of the various systems—nervous, circulatory, pulmonary, musculoskeletal, endocrine, gastrointestinal, genitourinary, or skin. However, certain accompanying symptoms may point to the primary system involved as follows:

Nervous: headache, dizziness, insomnia, irritability, nervousness, tremors, loss of sensation, ringing in the ears, deafness, visual disturbances, altered taste or smell.

Circulatory: chest pain or leg pain on exertion, shortness of breath, dizziness (especially in older persons), leg swelling during the day, pallor.

Pulmonary: cough, shortness of breath, chest pain, wheezing.

Musculoskeletal: aches and pains, joint swelling or tenderness, muscle weakness on exertion.

Endocrine: obesity (occasionally), headache and dizziness, sallow complexion, fatigue promptly relieved by sugar intake (morning Coke).

Gastrointestinal: prolonged nausea, vomiting, diarrhea, abdominal pain, loss of appetite, weight loss, jaundice.

Genitourinary: burning on urination, urinary frequency, flank pain or back pain at rib level, urgency, bloody or smoky urine.

Dermatologic: chronic skin eruptions, change in skin color, irritated moles or moles changing in size or color, itching, change in skin texture and pigmentation.

Physiologic Fatigue

The physical fatigue which results from natural physiologic processes is a good fatigue. It is a fatigue which tells the body that it is time to refuel and recuperate. It is body language that bespeaks the need for restoration of depleted reserves. For example, no one need tell the marathon runner who has just finished a twenty-six-mile run that it is time to rest and time to take on food and fluid.

What is the mechanism of physiologic fatigue? Muscular action demands a ready and constant supply of oxygen and fuel—glucose and fats. If the muscular activity is brief and intense—a sprint of perhaps two minutes or less—the respiratory system is unable to supply free oxygen fast enough to support the metabolic demands of the involved muscle. Thus the muscle obtains "free" energy in anaerobic fashion from a rapid breakdown of glycogen, a complex carbohydrate which yields glucose and subsequently lactic acid. In such activity large oxygen debts are incurred, and lactic acid accumulates in the blood. The fatigue which follows immediately after such bursts of all-out activity tends to disappear as the oxygen debt is repaid.

When the activity is more moderate and prolonged, as in distance running, this anaerobic energy production is operative for only a brief period of initial adjustment. After this period oxygen consumption rises to a new equilibrium-level that remains constant during the period of aerobic work and drops quickly to resting levels after the work is stopped. The intensity and quantity of fatigue which results from a given bit of muscular endeavor varies with the intensity and the duration of that endeavor, other factors being equal. In general the more intense and prolonged the endeavor, the greater the oxygen debt created, and the greater the accumulation of muscle metabolites that must be removed from the body before the pre-exercise state can be re-established.

The transformation of body fuels into energy is a highly complicated, cyclic process involving several different systems—phosphate, glucose-glycogen, citrate—and processes such as hydrogenation, oxidation, condensation, and decarboxylation, which require catalytic compounds known as enzymes and coenzymes. The reader doesn't have to be a physiologist, it is enough to say that physiologic fatigue is the state which speaks first of an oxygen debt, and next of the need for elimination of metabolic by-products and the replenishment of the fuel supply. In other words, it is a state which can be readily reversed by appropriate rest, food, and fluid. It is unfortunate that chronic fatigue of types other than physiologic is not so readily dealt with. In another sense, the most successful means of dealing with any type of chronic fatigue, as you shall see, is to reduce it to this most basic of forms, the physiologic one.

Mental Fatigue

Pure mental fatigue is a state next door to sleep. If you can understand what produces sleep, you can understand what produces mental fatigue. As it turns out, however, this Shakespearian balm that "knits up the ravelled sleeve of care" is as complex an entity as the brain itself. The airplane pilot with years of experience under his belt, flying a routine, uncomplicated flight may, on reaching his assigned altitude and setting the plane on automatic, be faced with pure mental fatigue. So may the student reading a dull assignment or the automobile driver speeding along a smooth, four-lane highway. What each of these must fight the hardest is falling asleep. Sleep is the natural antidote for this problem, curiously wrought as it is of such ingredients as boredom, routine, lack of interest, and monotony. But inject an element of risk, or of threat, or of necessity, and pure mental fatigue takes on emotional aspects.

If the tired pilot flies into a storm and his skill and mettle are called into play, he is no longer tired. If the nodding student, poring over his boring text, suddenly is told that he will be quizzed on the material tomorrow, he wakes up. If the sleepy driver speeding along the highway suddenly runs into a rainstorm and skids perilously close to a collision, his fatigue suddenly takes flight. Thus mental fatigue is that curious state of rather inanimate suspense just short of sleep which, like sleep, is capable of sudden reversal by a threat to the emotional security of the subject—in short, by arousal of the body's mechanism for fight or flight.

In asking why one becomes mentally fatigued, you might as well inquire: What makes one sleepy? The answer to this question is far from obvious.* Is it a result of diminished blood supply to the brain? It is now known that the volume of blood supplied to the brain under differing circumstances varies very little, although it is conceivable that there may be a shunting of blood from one part of the brain to another during sleep, with resultant affectation of consciousness centers through alterations in pressure, oxygen supply, carbon dioxide buildup, and the like. The recent evidence is that cerebral blood flow actually increases slightly during sleep and that oxygen consumption remains essentially unchanged.

Might it be that the body produces some chemical agent that is sleep inducing? Or is sleep a response to the buildup of "fatigue toxins?" And if so, why doesn't everyone jump out of bed in the A.M. raring to go? Carbon dioxide builds up in the blood during sleep, but is this cause or effect?

What of the endocrine system? Is sleep a downbeat of the pituitary gland's circadian rhythm? If so, then why doesn't removal of the pituitary gland lead to permanent sleep or wakefulness? It does neither.

In recent years, certain neuro-transmitters between the lower brain, or hypothalamus, and the pituitary gland have been shown to be essential to wakefulness. The production of such chemicals, within the brain tissue itself, is dependent on certain enzymes which play a catalytic role in the synthesis of one compound from a precursor or the breakdown of a substance into its precursor. Dopamine, adrenalin, and noradrenalin are such neurotransmitters. These same chemicals are manufactured by the adrenal gland in response to stress, so that if wakefulness is a product of such chemicals, then mental fatigue or sleep may, in a sense, represent a reversal of the process. Might sleepiness represent a deficiency of such hormones at nerve endings? It is all too well known that adrenalin, whether injected via a vein or produced by the adrenal gland in response to a threatening stimulus, is a powerful antidote to mental fatigue, as illustrated above. Very likely the truth of the matter lies somewhere in this very complicated realm.

Some have viewed sleep as the "original and basic state of life,"† noting that the fetus sleeps throughout its habitation of the womb, and that the growing infant and child sleep unless aroused by needful stimuli—a need to eat. In this early phase of life wakefulness is but a temporary interruption of sleep. Thus one might argue that when there is no cause to stay awake, one reverts to his natural state—sleep. Thus sleep, and not wakefulness, is the

*Roche Laboratories, *The Anatomy of Sleep* (Nutley, N.J.: Hoffmann-La-Roche, Inc., 1966). By permission.

†W.V. Cnuden, "A Study of Wake: An Approach to the Problems of Insomnia," *The Lancet* 1 (1957): 579.

natural state, and the ceesation of arousal—whether it be for survival or for pleasure—leads to sleep.

It follows, then, that whatever arouses leads away from sleep or mental fatigue, and that mental fatigue or sleep is the result of cessation of arousal. What all this boils down to is that when the adrenals and the nervous system cease to turn out the arousal hormones like adrenalin and noradrenalin in sufficient quantity to offset the natural state, sleep or mental fatigue results.

The essential difference, for example, in a tired pilot and a wide-awake one is a storm that has awakened his adrenals. The same is true of the student who discovers he is going to be tested on what he is reading, or the driver who skidded too close to the guardrail.

Hence the purely mentally fatigued individual may be viewed as one whose arousal mechanism is being challenged little or none, and whose neuro-transmitter hormones are, for one or another reason, functioning at a very low level.

Emotional Fatigue: The Tension-Fatigue Syndrome

No attempt is made here to explain the mechanisms of the depressions. Suffice it to say that genetics, environmental, neurochemical, and situational factors are involved, and that although much is known about depressions, exact mechanisms remain an enigma. That the balance between certain groups of neuro-transmitters is intricately involved seems true. But precisely how and why? In families where tendencies to depression exist, exactly what is transmitted? Or what is not? At any rate, the overall picture seems to indicate a preponderance of cholinergic activity in certain centers of the brain. Cholinergic activity, as you shall see, favors inertia, inactivity, and a subnormal level of physiologic functions. As stated earlier, the psychotic depressions—manic-depressives and endogenous types—account for a relatively small percentage of the huge bulk of emotional fatigue. Moreover, true psychoses call for expert psychiatric care.

Primarily, this book is concerned with the nonpsychotic, motivationally and environmentally derived type of fatigue, the type most commonly represented by the patient who confronts the doctor with the "I'm tired all the time" list of complaints. This I refer to as the chronic-fatigue, or tension-fatigue, syndrome. To be sure, there is a great deal of genetic, environmental, neurochemical, and neuroendocrine involvement here, perhaps as much as in the depressions, but of a different quality and quantity. You cannot hope to become an expert in any of these fields in so short a space. But because tension-fatigue is inextricably linked to chronic stress, it is essential to your understanding of chronic tension-fatigue that you become familiar with certain basic concepts at this point: (1) stress, (2) tension, (3) Selye's general adaptation syndrome (G.A.S.), and (4) the fight-or-flight response of Castle.

Some Basics

Stress. In the biologic sense, stress is that force, of either external or internal origin, which threatens the peaceful status quo of the organism. It may by physical, mental, or emotional in its primary context. A lion cub suckling at its mother's breast has food, warmth, and security. It is at peace with its environment. It is under no stress. But if it wanders from the pride and is suddenly confronted with a predatory antagonist, its security and indeed its very life are threatened. The situation becomes stressful and the fight-or-flight mechanism (which is considered momentarily) is triggered to provide relief.

Most human beings arrive at various stages of life through encountering stress and relieving it through some variant of the fight-or-flight process. For example, when the baby becomes hungry—a form of stress—he cries (fights verbally) and obtains food; by this process he grows. The schoolchild, through the stress of study, grows mentally and at length is able to take his place in society. Each examination and each assignment is a threat to his level of knowledge, his momentary status quo; he can meet such recurring threats either by standing and fighting or by running away. Likewise, the aspiring bank teller, with his eye on the bank presidency, eventually arrives at this goal, if successful, by accepting challenge after challenge to his status quo, or even his very security. He may find himself in a situation where he would like to run, but if he is to succeed, he must stand and fight. Each time that a life situation demands a change, or threatens security, or disturbs the tranquility of an individual, stress is the result. In our society the ultimate test of manhood is how successfully a person copes with stress.

First you must know terms connected with stress. The *stressor* is the agent responsible for the stress. For example, to a person lost in a snowstorm, cold is the stressor agent. To a football lineman the opposing players are the stressor agents. To a fireman a conflagration is responsible for the stress; to a physician the disease process that threatens his patient. And so on. There are many different types of stressor agents: (1) physical ones such as extremes of heat or cold; (2) physiological ones such as deficiencies of oxygen, food, or water; (3) pathological ones such as disease states; (4) mental ones such as problems relating to your occupation or to confrontation with a gigantic mental task; and (5) emotional ones such as relate to family problems, finances, occupational problems, or health. The *stress* resulting from the stressor agent is that force, or combination of forces, acting upon the *stressee*, or stress recipient.

Loop a rubber band around each of your two middle fingers and put the band on stretch by moving your hands apart. You have created a fairly accurate picture of stress. The *stressor* in this instance is the fingers to which the band is attached. The *stress* applied is the force necessary to move the hands a certain distance apart. And the *stressee* is the rubber band itself. If the hands are moved apart, say one foot, the resultant stress is not nearly so great as if moved apart twice or three times that distance; the amount of stress is proportional to the force applied by the stressor agent. Again, the amount of stress capable of being applied by a given stressor is directly proportional to the strength of the stressor.

Let's consider our lion cub again for a moment. Suppose that the antagonist it encounters outside the fold is a small rodent. While it may frighten him somewhat if he has never seen one before, it is certainly not a threat to his ultimate security. But suppose that he encounters a hungry hyena. Here is a large, strong threat which is capable of applying considerably more stress than the small rodent. An analogy exists here to life situations. John needs ten dollars to purchase some groceries ordered by his wife, but he forgets his wallet. He is confronted with a minor stress situation in which the stressor is the need for cash, the stress is the discomfort of *dis*tress caused him when he must break the news of his absent-mindedness to his wife, and he is, of course, the *stressee.* But consider John the next day when he finds that his tax bill is two thousand dollars greater than he had anticipated, and he is overdrawn at the bank. The resultant stress is considerably greater because greater sums are involved with far less flexible people—the solution demands considerably greater effort.

In general, the greater the ease with which a given threat can be removed, or security restored, the less potent the stressor agent. A person overheated in a hot office may solve his problem by turning on a fan or an air-conditioner. But a person lost on a desert is faced with a problem of quite a different magnitude—excessive heat. The traffic-controller at a small airport is faced with the same type of problem that one is at a major airport, but the magnitude is as different as the size of a Piper Cub and a 727 jet.

Stressor agents make demands on the stressee. It is the size and duration of these demands which determine the amount of stress imposed. Talking down an airplane through a ceiling zero storm creates stress, but talking down ten of them multiplies the stress considerably. Or fighting a two-alarm fire for one hour may be stressful, but fighting a four-alarm blaze for many hours is considerably more so.

Thus, stress possesses the attributes of intensity (quality) and duration (quantity). And the greater the magnitude of either or both of these factors, the greater the total stress. Thus a small rubber band put on a six-inch stretch for six minutes would return without difficulty to its previous length and shape. But a band stretched to a length of sixteen inches for six minutes would not do so, nor would a band stretched to a length of six inches for sixty minutes. This is to say that stress, if of sufficient intensity or duration, may irretrievably alter the stressee. Consider an example. Suppose that Jane discovers that her son is having grade trouble. When it is discovered, after proper investigation, that his problem relates to a visual defect readily corrected with a pair of glasses, the resultant stress is short-lived and abruptly terminated. There are no irreversible effects. But suppose instead that the boy's problem is due to involvement with drugs. And suppose, further, that the boy's father is deceased. Now the stress on Jane is multiplied many times, and the resultant tension-fatigue considerably more intense and of a more enduring nature. Before the problem is solved, Jane's tension and fatigue are likely to produce irreversible damage to her psyche and soma.

It becomes axiomatic that great stress—stress of great intensity or long duration—produces great tension-fatigue. In a given individual, there is a somewhat linear relationship between the two. As you shall see, however, the same stress produces different degrees of tension-fatigue in different persons, a result of different genes and different environments.

Tension. Tension is the resultant composite change in certain physiologic parameters—muscle tone, blood pressure, heart rate, pupil size, and so on—which the stressee experiences as a result of stress. The stretched rubber band is smaller in thickness and may vibrate tunefully when plucked while on stretch, manifestations of changes in its physical state—tension. This is an important concept, for in the biologic organism, many harmful (and fatiguing) chemical changes accompany the physical ones manifested as tension. The relationship to fatigue becomes readily apparent when you consider subsequently Selye's G.A.S. and Castle's fight-or-flight mechanism as it applies to civilized man. These are discussed shortly.

Autonomic Nervous System. The autonomic nervous system is, as the name implies, that portion of the nervous system which functions autonomously—independently of volition*—and no one can intelligently study stress, the G.A.S., or fight-or-flight without considering it. It is responsible, in large measure, for the regulation of heart rate, blood pressure, pupil size, sweating, body temperature, blood-vessel size, muscle tone, digestive activities, and the like. It is composed of two major components—the *sympathetic*, whose fibers originate mainly in the spinal cord, and the *parasympathetic*, whose fibers emanate chiefly from the brain stem and the end segment of the cord, as shown in Figure 3. The table on page 39 lists the basic functions of the two components of the system.

Note that the sympathetic portion of the system causes, in general, an elevation in the various physiologic functions such as heart rate, pulse rate, and respiration, whereas the parasympathetic portion causes a lowering of these same functions. Stimulation of the sympathetics is thus comparable to the effect of an injection of adrenalin, such that the sympathetics play the dominant role in readying an organism for fight or flight.

Originating in the lower brain, the hypothalamus, the autonomic system has endings all over the body—in blood vessels, lungs, heart, kidneys, adrenals, the gastrointestinal tract, and sweat glands. Its tie-in with the endocrine system (a group of glands which secrete hormones into the bloodstream) enables it to work in concert with liver, pancreas, thyroid, and adrenals in regulating the supply of body fuels in times of stress, when fight or flight is at hand.

*Recent studies of biofeedback mechanisms indicate that the autonomic system (despite its name) is indeed subject to volitional alteration.

AUTONOMIC NERVOUS SYSTEM

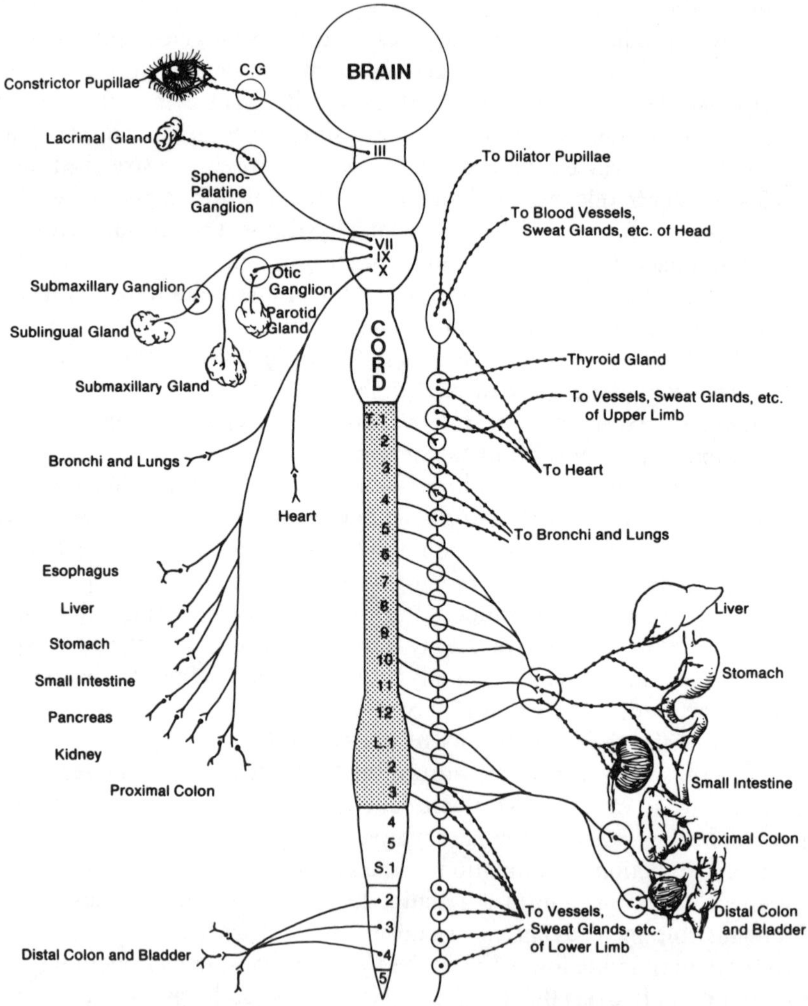

*Figure 3.** The parasympathetic outflow is represented to the left, the sympathetic outflow to the right of the brain and spinal cord (center band). See text.

* From Chas. H. Best and Norman B. Taylor, *The Physiological Basis of Medical Practice,* (Baltimore: Williams and Wilkins, 1945). Reprinted with permission.

A COMPARISON OF SYMPATHETIC AND PARASYMPATHETIC INFLUENCE ON BODY FUNCTIONS*

Body Function	Under Sympathetic Influence (Sympathotonia, Adrenergic Preponderance)	Under Parasympathetic Influence (Vagatonia, Cholinergic Preponderance)
Heart rate	Increased	Decreased
Blood pressure	Increased	Decreased
Muscle tension	Increased	Decreased
Cardiac output	Increased	Decreased
Respiratory rate and depth	Increased	Decreased
Glandular and metabolic activity	Increased	Decreased
Anticipatory response (readiness for action)	Stimulated	Dampened
Fight-or-flight response	Aided	Hindered
Exertion	Aided	Hindered
Restoration (sleep and rest)	Hindered	Aided

Note that the sympathetic nervous system is, in general, one which speeds up body functions and increases metabolic demands, whereas the reverse is true of the parasympathetic system. Normally these two systems are finely balanced, each complementing the other. But prolonged (chronic) stress or frequently repeated episodes of acute stress, such as commonly result from present-day, high-pressure living, causes unrelenting stimulation of the sympathetic system, with resultant adrenergic preponderance, unless an outlet, such as exercise, is provided. Such sympathetic preponderance promotes numerous stress-related diseases. The net result of exercise is promotion of parasympathetic influence (vagatonia) and inhibition of sympathetic influence (sympathotonia), apparently through maximal, periodic stimulation of the sympathetics. Thus the fundamental effect of exercise is to restore balance between these two finely tuned counterparts of the nervous system.

* From M.F. Graham, M.D., *Prescription for Life,* (New York: McKay, 1966). Reprinted with permission.

In essence, a major function of the autonomic nervous system is to maintain the integrity of body-defense mechanisms, wherein the sympathetics are the pathways of action, and the parasympathetics are the pathways of recuperation—restoration and rest.

G.A.S. of Selye. Over three decades ago a Canadian physiologist by the name of Hans Selye described what he refers to as the *general adaptation syndrome* (G.A.S.).* Although revised and refined since its first description, the original concept has remained essentially unchanged. It is based on the tenet that biologic stress is met by an increase in gland size and in the discharge of adrenal-gland (stress-gland) compounds. These compounds are known as *corticoids* and are produced in the cortex of the adrenal gland. See Figure 4.

When an organism is exposed to a stressor agent, the resultant stress, according to Selye, causes a nonspecific, three-stage physiologic response:

1. The *alarm reaction* (AR) occurs in two phases: shock and countershock.

In the *shock phase* the organism is dealt a "haymaker" to those mechanisms which regulate body temperature, blood pressure, muscle tone, blood concentration, and various chemical balances in the blood. For the most part such processes are depressed, or lowered, such that if the initial insult is great enough, death may ensue. Varying from minutes to hours in duration, shock always develops rapidly, affects the entire body (is systemic), and is intense. Numerous stressor agents may precipitate shock, among them trauma, hemorrhage, burns, cold, heat, irradiation, emotional stress, muscular exercise, asphyxia, infection, drugs and toxins, diet, and even bed rest. The shock incitor strikes decisively and rapidly, like an uppercut swung from the floor and landing on the "button." So intense and so swift is its onset that there is no time for the adrenal glands to rise to the defense. Hence the overall picture of depressed body functions, lowered blood pressure, lowered body temperature, loss of muscle tone, altered consciousness, and so on.

Following immediately on the heels of the shock phase is the phase of *countershock*. Here reversal of the shock phase begins. Body defenses are garnered and slowly rise to the occasion. The adrenal cortex, under the influence of the hypothalamus and pituitary, increases its production of hormones, blood pressure rises, blood volume increases, body temperature rises toward normal, and blood chemistry values normalize. Slowly the kayoed boxer gets to his knees, shakes his head, and prepares to enter the fray.

2. The *stage of resistance* is but an extension of the countershock phase of the AR. In this stage an excessive production of adrenal corticoids may cause an overreaction to the stressor agent, characterized by sustained elevations in blood pressure (hypertension), blood sugar (diabetes), and immune complexes playing a causative role in many degenerative diseases. Thus have

*Hans Selye, *Stress of Life*, rev. ed. (New York: McGraw-Hill, 1976). Reprinted with permission.

THE ADRENAL GLANDS

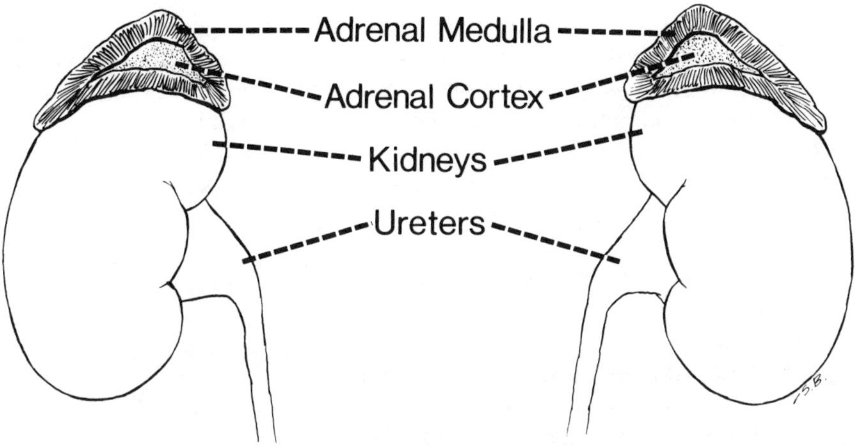

*Figure 4:** Each adrenal gland is in reality two glands in one, and the medulla is not properly a gland at all, but a converted, specialized group of cells belonging to the sympathetic nervous system (Figure 3).

The *medulla* secretes the catechols epinephrine (adrenalin) and norepinephrine (noradrenalin), so essential to fight or flight, though, perhaps paradoxically, not essential to life. Whereas the generalized effect of norepinephrine is that of constriction of blood vessels, it dilates the coronary arteries. The drug does not increase heart rate or force, and its increase of peripheral resistance causes a rise in blood pressure which reflexly slows the heart and tends to decrease cardiac output. Epinephrine increases heart rate and force of contraction, with resultant increase in cardiac output, and dilates blood vessels in certain organs, notably liver and skeletal muscle. Both epinephrine and norepinephrine, but chiefly the former, cause a rise in blood glucose. Both mobilize certain fats and, acting in conjunction with thyroid and adrenal cortical secretions, increase the rate of metabolism.

The *cortex*, chiefly under the influence of ACTH (adrenocorticotrophic hormone) from the pituitary gland, secretes a group of complex compounds known as steroids. The glucocorticoid steroids primarily affect carbohydrate and protein metabolism, the mineralocorticoid steroids salt and fluid balance, and the sex hormones primarily reproductive functions (to a minor extent).

* From M.F. Graham, M.D., *Prescription for Life,* (New York: McKay, 1966). Reprinted with permission.

such diseases as essential hypertension and stomach ulcers, for example, been labeled diseases of adaptation, inasmuch as the stage of resistance represents an adaptive response of the organism to stress. More is said of this later.

The stage of resistance represents the sum total of the various systemic physiologic reactions to a stressor agent to which the organism has adapted, and is characterized by increased resistance to that agent and a decreased resistance to other stressor stimuli. For example, repeated exposure to extreme cold renders that organism more resistant to cold, but less resistant to extreme heat, which is to say that adaptability to one stressor agent may be gained at the expense of decreased resistance to others. In this stage the floored and groggy boxer has risen to his full height, cleared his sensorium, and launched a counterattack.

3. The *stage of exhaustion* is characterized by a downward turn in the various parameters to which I have referred (blood pressure, body temperature, blood volume, etc.) until they approach or surpass, though more slowly, the values seen in the initial shock phase.

Weeks or months of repeated hammering away at an organism by stressful stimuli causes a breakdown in adaptability, so that resistance begins to crumble. Even the toughest of organisms cannot indefinitely endure a potent stressor agent. Under the influence of continuous adaptive maneuvers, the "adaptation energy" of the organism is eventually exhausted, and resistance once again gives way to chronic shock, or exhaustion.

In this stage our heroic boxer becomes rubber-legged. It is the last round and he has fought long and hard, but his opponent is too dogged, too massive, too inexorable. And so at length he goes down beneath the incessant blows.

The G.A.S. of Selye is but a series of stages through which an organism subjected to stress—any systemic stress—passes on the road to adapting to that stress. The greater the stress, the greater the response, and the more repetitively any given stimulus is applied, the more specific the response to that stimulus becomes. Any systemic stress can cause very similar general manifestations, and an overresponse to a given stress factor may in itself result in a disease of adaptation. Typical of such diseases are emotional disturbances, headaches, insomnia, gastrointestinal upsets, high blood pressure, and certain types of rheumatic or allergic disorders, as well as cardiovascular and kidney disease. The G.A.S. is general in its nature, adaptive in its purpose, and is composed of a broad collection of responses centered around the adrenal cortex and its hormones.

Fight or Flight. The crackle of twigs outside the cave entrance caused a group of physiologic reactions in the body of the caveman within. His pupils dilated, his pulse quickened, his blood pressure heightened, his muscles tensed. What awaited him in the darkness—friend or foe? If friend, there was no problem. But if foe—sabertooth or enemy tribesman—then his body was prepared to meet the threat by either of two alternatives: fighting or fleeing. As shown in Figure 5 the preparation for fight or flight is mediated through

THE FIGHT-OR-FLIGHT (ADRENERGIC) RESPONSE

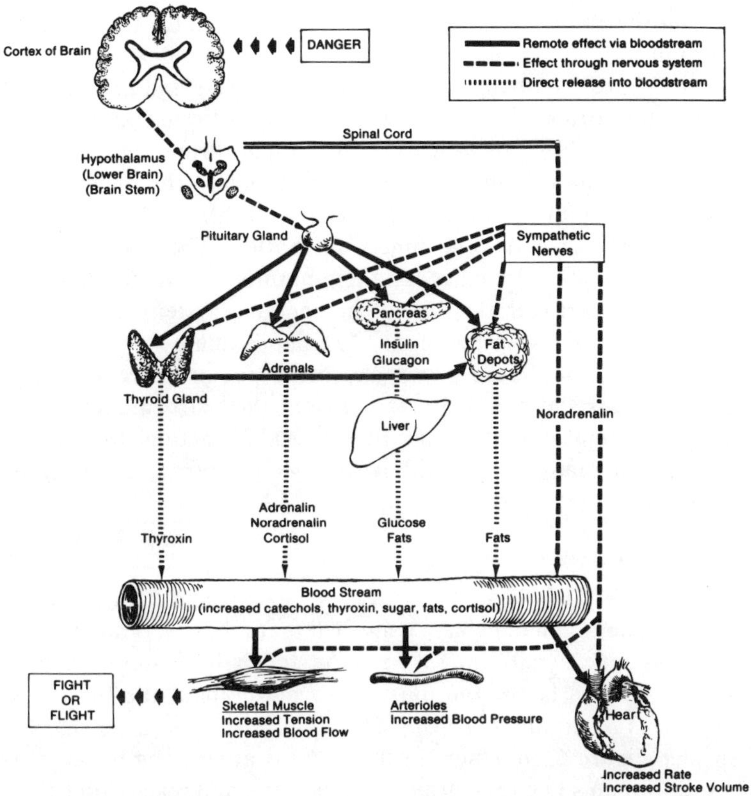

*Figure 5:** This response is a complex, primitive one in which the body is physiologically prepared to do battle with, or to flee, an imminent danger. Under the influence of the nervous system, the endocrine glands release the necessary materials into the bloodstream, with a resultant increase in blood pressure, heart rate, muscle tension, and flow of blood to the skeletal muscles in particular. The normal means of releasing the stored-up tension resulting from this "adrenergic" response is through the skeletal muscles – through exercise. When such release is habitually not available to the body, diseases due to stress – such as ulcers, high blood pressure, and cardiovascular disease (see text) – may eventually result. Modern-day tensions of living produce the same overall effect as external dangers, but modern civilization denies man the fight-or-flight release, except through exercise.

* From M.F. Graham, M.D., *Prescription for Life,* (New York: McKay, 1966). Reprinted with permission.

the nervous and endocrine systems, and again the adrenal glands play a key role. In fact, such preparation is comparable in terms of body response to the alarm (countershock) and resistance stages of adaptation. It represents an isolated component, in time, of the general adaptation syndrome. In effect, it zeroes in on the initial phases of adaptation as it relates to response to a single stimulus.

Note in Figure 5 that the stimulation of endocrine and nervous systems originates in the cortex of the brain, which in turn is turned on by the danger which represents a threat to security or status quo. From these higher brain centers, the message is transmitted to lower centers—the hypothalamus—which, acting in conjunction with the pituitary, or "master" gland, pulls the switches that set the entire machinery in motion. The various endocrine glands, especially the adrenal, pour their hormones into the bloodstream and, acting in concert with the sympathetic nervous system, cause a buildup of fuel—sugar and fats—in the blood. The pupils dilate to aid and abet vision, hearing becomes more acute, the heart pumps more vigorously in response to the adrenalin, blood pressure rises, the heart rate increases, and muscle tone is heightened in preparation for sudden action. In short the entire body is made ready to "get with it" or "get away from it," whatever the threat may be.

Strife-Goal Concept

What does this diatribe about stress, the G.A.S., and fight or flight have to do with fatigue? I can tell you in a nutshell that it has everything to do with the chronic-fatigue syndrome so common to civilized man. In order to understand why this is so, you must know more about the fight in which modern man is so commonly involved.

Consider Figure 6, in which a subject (S) is attempting to reach a goal (G). In order to do so he must leave from point A and reach point B. Along the way he may encounter one or more obstacles (O), and he must contend with the environment (E). The ease with which S reaches the goal is determined by a number of interacting factors:

Factors intrinsic to S:

1. Physical makeup
2. Physical status (state of health)
3. Stage of growth
4. Past experience
5. Mental-emotional makeup (personality)
6. Training
7. Age and sex
8. Ethnic background

Factors peculiar to G:

1. Desirability
2. Definition (vague versus clear-cut, concrete versus abstract)
3. Complexity

THE GOAL-STRIFE CONCEPT OF FATIGUE

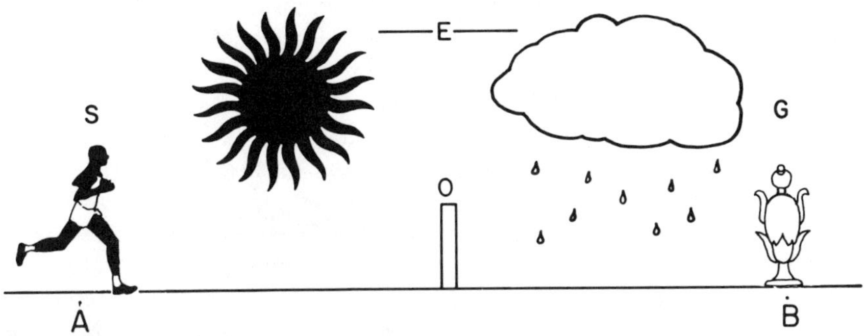

Figure 6: In the diagram, S represents the subject, G the goal, E the environment, and O the obstacle(s) encountered as S, starting from point A, strives to reach goal G at point B. The total fatigue generated by this effort is the sum total of factors inherent and acquired in the subject, the proximity and complexity of the goal, the number and size of the obstacle(s) encountered along the way, and whether the environment is smooth and friendly or rough and hostile.

Thus the composite cause of chronic fatigue in any given person may be vastly different from that in another individual, since subjects, goals, environment, and obstacles are never precisely the same from one instance to the next.

Obstacles between A and B (number, size, type, acute or chronic)
Environment:

1. Physical aspects
2. Emotional aspects (friendly or hostile, cheerful or depressing, etc.)
3. Complexity

Let's take a brief look at each of these major ingredients:

The Subject. Just as it is easier for a 6 feet 10 inches forward to dunk a basket in a game of basketball than it is for a five-tenner to do so, so it is that any given individual may deal with a given life situation easier than another. Thus when considering the amount of stress produced in a person by a given environmental situation, it is essential to consider certain characteristics of the subject.

1. Physical makeup. Nowhere is the role of physical makeup in the strife-goal concept better illustrated than in the realm of athletic endeavor. The long, tall individual may be somewhat of a freak in the workaday world, but on the basketball court he is king. Or the 300-pound, 6-feet 8-inch hulk of humanity may feel out of place in the midst of midgets in the classroom, but on the football field he is a bulwark in the defensive line.

Physical traits are important in the business world as well. The larger person often innately feels and exudes more self-confidence, and whereas he must be looked up to physically, he creates an aura of being looked up to mentally as well. Thus it is that physically big people are more often found in leadership positions.

But in certain occupations small people may have an advantage, for example, the horse-racing jockey. And round men make the best Santa Clauses.

The presence or absence of distinctive features—curly hair, a well-formed face or profile, good body proportions—play an important role not only in what avenues in life a person may pursue, but also in his formation of a pleasing body image in his own mind. A person pleased with his personal physical appearance and makeup is much more likely to be a confident individual than one who has a poor body image of himself.

Mary was a college girl who had been successful in whatever pursuit she undertook. She was attractive, but she became obsessed with the idea that her thighs were out of proportion to the rest of her body. (They were not dramatically out of proportion.) She placed herself on a self-imposed diet, a poor approach to her exaggerated problem, with resultant overall weight loss and physical fatigue, such that all areas of her life suffered as a consequence. Previously a good student, she became a poor one. Once a good athlete, she became second-rate. Once very popular with other students, she became an object of pity. Only expert psychiatric intervention restored her, over a protracted period, to a semblance of her former self. Most individuals suffer from some flaw, albeit minor, in body image. It is the rare person who likes all of what he sees of himself. Mary was an extreme example of what happens to most people, because of a lack of self-acceptance, to a far less drastic degree.

Your physical makeup—large or small, beautiful or ugly, whole or deformed, well-proportioned or poorly so—is your most visible and readily appraised equipment in the strife of life. Small wonder that it plays a major role in success or failure—and thus in tension and fatigue production.

2. Physical status. The person who is chronically ill, or who has a body deformity or handicap, must make his pass at life with an albatross about his neck. Some few convert such a liability into an asset. A doctor developed a severe spinal deformity as a result of polio in childhood. Instead of being mentally as well as physically victimized by the disease, he became determined to study medicine. And study it he did, becoming an expert in the field of care of polio victims in the days before polio vaccine eradicated the disease.

Unfortunately, most handicapped persons do not react so favorably. They fall prey to self-pity. There are numerous sources of help for the bodily handicapped today, and there is no reason that such individuals cannot rechannel their thought processes into productive and highly satisfying fields of endeavor.

3. Stage of growth. The imposition of a given task or workload on an individual before he is mature may place him at a distinct disadvantage. This applies to physical or mental or emotional maturity. The seventeen-year-old tennis player may be a champion in her own age bracket, but pit her against more mature players and she becomes an also-ran; what she needs is time to grow and develop. Similarly, the teacher confronted with teaching a given course may, with only an AB degree, be severely handicapped; but with an MA or PhD no problem exists. What is needed is further mental growth. In a tense, chronically fatigued individual, it is important to know whether he has been thrust into a life situation before he was far enough along in his growth to adequately cope with it.

4. *Past experience*. Past experience is a part of mental or emotional growth, and thus relates to the stage of growth (as above). The most desirable characteristic in a potential employee, other factors being equal, is experience. The actual performance of a task begets confidence, and confidence in turn begets smoother performance. Thus the neophyte in any given situation may commonly experience tension and fatigue, which disappear as experience and confidence develop.

5. *Mental-emotional makeup* (personality). A person begins life with certain genetically predetermined personality traits, just as it is predetermined that he will have blue eyes or black hair. Some persons are innately high-strung, some innately sedate and phlegmatic. Such traits may be guided, but they can never be changed. A good (desirable) set of such traits makes it much easier for that person to cope with circumstance. The calm, confident individual with an icy-veined mien is, in the presence of pressure or crisis, much less likely to be a victim of chronic tension and fatigue than the person who pushes the panic button at the slightest provocation. While training and experience can do much to improve the overt manifestations of an innately tense individual, such a person will, at least in his sympathetic nervous system, always tend to react in hyper fashion to a tense situation. Here again there is no substitute for a good set of genes.

6. *Training*. Dr. Young was a good general practitioner, but when the opportunity came to join a group of surgeons, he found himself required to do surgery for which he had never received specific training. Though he performed it well, he was under constant tension for fear he would make an error.

Many psychiatrists feel that every individual has his own "break point," beyond which a given stress will result in a malfunction of the personality. An example might be ten men in a trench on the front lines in WWI. On the signal to go over the top, two of the men might faint dead away, four might be out of the trench immediately on command, and four might have to be prodded into action. The stress reaction of any one person in a given situation is thus a reflection of background, personality, and experience, as variegated as there are individuals. Since, as you shall see, fatigue is a byproduct of stress, it likewise bears a proportionate relationship to the intrinsic qualities of the individual involved.

7. *Age and sex*. A woman may find herself in a job previously held only

by men. Though she may be perfectly capable, her associates continually watch for her to commit an error, thus creating needless tension. Similarly, an older person may suddenly assume the position of a younger one; in trying to prove that older people still make good employees, he is subconsciously striving unnecessarily to prove himself.

8. Ethnic background. Racial and language barriers may produce obstacles that increase stress proportionately. Dr. Kay, for example, may possess all the qualifications necessary to fill a certain medical post, but he is unable to speak fluently the language required. Therefore he finds himself under considerable tension that would not otherwise exist.

The Goal. A goal is an objective toward which one directs attention, time, energy, and resources until it is either reached or abandoned. It may relate to a person, a place, or a thing, or it may be an idealistic intangible, such as power, recognition, or fame.

Goals may be categorized according to the area of life to which they primarily relate.

1. Job
2. Money (wealth)
3. Family
4. Health
5. Security
6. Leisure activity
7. Training (education, skill development)
8. Recognition
9. Position (social, academic, etc.)

Obviously multiple goals may exist, either in the same or in different categories. The assignment of priorities to goals is of extreme importance.

Goals may also be categorized as to immediacy, that is as to short-term, intermediate, or long-term. The tenure placed upon each of these is arbitrary and varies with the age, background, and training of the individual.

Still another classification refers to the rank of importance assigned to a goal, that is, its priority.

The complete classification of a goal would entail its recognition as to:

1. Immediacy (short-term, intermediate, long-term)
2. Primary area of life involved (job, family, social, financial, etc.)
3. Priority (A, B, C, etc.)

Goals also possess individual attributes, such as desirability, proximity, elusiveness, concreteness, complexity, and the like. Let's take a look at some of these.

1. Desirability. A highly desirable and worthwhile goal is far less likely to produce fatigue than is one of lesser worth, presumably because the motivation is greater. A good yardstick with which to measure this attribute of a goal is social acceptability. A preposterous, but lucid, example would be

Carol's working and saving her money to buy a gun. If she purposes to use the gun to hunt or to protect her household, the goal is worthwhile; but if she intends to use the weapon to dispose of someone she violently dislikes, the goal is socially undesirable.

Such goals are filled with stress by their very nature. Joe wanted to make a lot a money because, as a boy raised in penurious circumstances, his father had made him work hard and had treated him very shabbily. When Joe had reached his goal, he soon gained the reputation of using his wealth to lord it over his associates, and he became generally disliked. Joe's real goal was ill-used power, and money was but his instrument. The purpose behind his goal was socially undesirable, and both its achievement and its realization caused untold stress, anxiety, and chronic fatigue in its seeker.

2. Proximity. Quite obviously, the more nearly within reach a goal, the less stressful it is. Any student will tell you that it is considerably easier to endure the rigors of a senior year in high school or college than it is those of the freshman one. The "at-handness" of the diploma or the degree is a powerful antidote for fatigue.

Contrariwise, the distant goal, especially if ill-defined or tenuous, is a source of much more stress and hence fatigue. Other factors being equal, there is, in fact, a direct relationship between the distance to the goal and the stress produced.

3. Elusiveness. Who could argue that it is easier (less stressful) to catch a tortoise than a greased pig? The hard-to-catch goal—one which constantly eludes the grasp or must be reached in a series of uncertain steps—is a real fatigue producer. The writer who, for example, has collected rejection slip after rejection slip over a period of years soon begins to think her goal slippery and unattainable, and fatigue may become her constant companion. In this regard, it is far less stressful to cope with a physical goal (with which one can come to tangible grips) than a mental-emotional one.

4. Concreteness. How readily definable is the goal? Is it abstract and difficult to conceive? Or can it be easily comprehended?

For example, the course prescribed for graduation from high school is straightforward and well-delineated, both as to time and content. But the course required to become a high political figure, for example president, is much more tenuous and loaded with the vagaries of circumstance.

The difference is comparable to that between a problem in mathematics, which can be solved by certain logical steps, and a problem in metaphysics, where many of the involved factors are difficult to define, much less to measure.

5. Complexity. Simple goals usually have simple solutions and are much less likely to foster tension and fatigue. The more complex and more involved a goal, the more difficult is its attainment. Hence the more tension and fatigue it is likely to beget in the subject striving to achieve it.

As an analogy, the road to a mountain peak, coursing through forests, over streams, and up rocky precipices, is considerably more fatiguing than a walk around the block. The more intricate the design of a carpet, the more difficult the weaving. Simplicity is the handmaiden of rest and complexity the factory of stress.

6. Realisticality. Is the goal realistic? Is it within the realm of possibility? of probability? The near-blind individual who loves flying and aspires to fly an aircraft is obviously setting an impossible goal. The man who has a $10,000 bank account and a $15,000 annual income would do far better to set his sights on a $50,000 piece of property than a $500,000 one. Facing up to facts—fitting the goal to the situation—is extremely important. All sorts of stress and its attendant bedfellows, anxiety and fatigue, are created by the incongruity of a goal and the actual set of circumstances. To be sure, one reads Horatio Alger stories of beating tremendous odds in this, that, or the other—setting records in spite of a physical handicap, zooming from rags to riches on a dime—but if you set goals from this viewpoint, you are playing the exception rather than the rule. It is comparable to putting your money on a twenty-to-one shot at the race track, as opposed to a repeat winner at three to two. If you win, you win big. But if you lose—and the odds are you will—you also lose big. In setting goals reality is of the utmost importance. Play the odds. Use your head, not your emotions. In the long run the payoff will be much, much greater and the stress created much, much less.

7. Clarity. Is the goal well-defined? clear-cut? Ill-defined, hazy goals do not permit clear thinking, and hazy thinking commonly results in disastrous and therefore stressful decisions. A very ready example is of a person sitting down to write a book without having made preparation as to outline or context. He has a clouded idea of the whole project, and perhaps a title. But when the blank page is attacked, what results is a meandering, meaningless conglomeration of words having neither direction nor meaning. The result can only be failure.

Jane wants to go into business for herself, but she doesn't know what kind or how much money, time, and effort are involved. She goes to the bank to borrow money, but naturally is refused because she hasn't thought her goal out in its entirety, if at all. This creates anxiety and frustration and destroys self-confidence. With a clearly-defined goal she could have avoided such stress.

Thus your objective—goal—may be a source of stress if it is: (1) too distant, (2) too large, (3) too unrealistic, (4) too nebulous (lacks clarity), (5) lacking in direction, (6) lacking in purpose, or (7) assigned the wrong priority.

Of course, it is basic to realize such qualities are relative to the individual under consideration. A goal too distant, too large, or too unrealistic for one person may not be at all distant for another. Incidentally, the same is true of environmental obstacles. A simple example would be that of a twelve-year-old football player who wants to try out for a professional football team. His goal is obviously too large and too unrealistic. But for a twenty-one-year-old Heisman Trophy winner, left behind in the draft, such a goal is not out of reason or reach. Of course, the twelve-year-old player may in time be perfectly capable of attaining such a goal, but for now it is too distant.

Environmental Obstacles. The terrain between you and a goal may be either readily traversable, with few obstacles, or it may be rife with obstacles that follow in rapid succession. For example, the sprinter's terrain is smooth and fast, while that of the marathon runner is uphill and down, and that of the hurdle jumper has a number of jumps interposed between starting point and finish.

The Environment. The physical and emotional aspects of the environment, as well as the simplicity or complexities of the environment, affect the individual.

1. Physical aspects. A hot, humid environment is much more inducive to fatigue than a cool, pleasant one. The greater the extremes of temperature, the less efficient are workers under such conditions. The air-conditioning of plants and schools, while considerably increasing the expense of operating such establishments, pays for itself in the long run many times over by increasing the efficiency of worker and student.

2. Emotional aspects (friendly or hostile). Friendly environments are constituted by a general atmosphere conducive to attainment of a goal. They are encouraging, positive, and tend to reenforce your drive and initiative.

On the other hand, hostile environments tend to thwart your desires and efforts. They are negative and antagonistic, and resist, rather than reenforce, movement toward a goal.

Environmental friendliness or hostility may refer to anything from room temperature or climate zone, to attitudes of fellow workers. Furthermore what may be a friendly environment for one type of undertaking may be hostile for another.

Mary was a freshman medical student studying anatomy at a table with several chauvinistic males. She was the butt of many jokes, inasmuch as her cohorts were, at least subconsciously, antagonistic to the idea of females studying medicine. She was constantly on guard, stressed by lack of acceptance. At her request, she was moved to a table where women were accepted into the group, and her tension eased considerably.

3. Environmental structure (simple or complex). Simplicity or complexity of an environment refers to the number and magnitude of friendly or antagonistic elements within it which are acting upon you at any given time. For example, extreme heat poses a problem for the marathon runner, but add to that excessive humidity and complete lack of a breeze, and the problem is compounded. Tom may be shooting for an executive position, constantly threatened by a fierce competitor, Bill. But add to that strife a sick mother who is his sole responsibility, and Tom's environment becomes complicated indeed.

Obviously simple environments, in which the number of forces to be dealt with at any one time are relatively few, are far less conducive to stress—and thus to tension-fatigue—than are environments loaded with stress factors, especially hostile ones.

A Summation. Under the concept of the G.A.S. adaptations to life situations represent the composite response to interacting forces originating from within you, from the environment, or from the goal. Such adaptation is as simple or as complex as any or all of these major components. In civilized societies, in particular, the interacting forces may be legion, so much so that it becomes difficult, if not impossible, to separate them one from another. And the more complex the composite picture, the more intense the generated stress, as a general rule, and the more chronic the tension and fatigue that accompany.

The Sams of this world (whom you will meet in a later chapter) are complex persons in a complex environment striving for complex goals. It is little wonder, when you consider all the factors, that so many are tense and fatigued most of the time.

The feeling known as chronic fatigue may be viewed as but the result of an ever-changing, almost kaleidoscopic interaction of you with your environment as you strive to attain a certain goal or goals (see Figure 6).

Recognition of Stress

Stress, that most important of all factors in emotional fatigue, is often endured simply because it is not recognized. Stress is, at least in our consideration here, any force which threatens to disrupt the continuity and security of a stable and satisfactory life pattern, or which interferes with the attainment of a desirable goal. "Stress (external force) yields tension (internal physiologic changes) yields chronic fatigue" is a fundamental concept.

In order to recognize stress, we must be aware of the various types of stress as to (1) content, and to (2) origin, or source.

Physical stress may originate from within or without. Stress from within may be due to illness or to a state of physical deprivation (as in starvation). Stress from without may relate to working conditions, conditions of climate, exposure to noxious materials, and so on. Again, there is no pure type of stress, which is to say that stress affecting primarily the physical, mental, or emotional aspect of an individual also affects the other aspects as well.

Mental stress may also originate from within or without. For example, the imposition of a huge "learning load"—required study for an important exam—represents mental stress from without. Stress from within originates from poor mental attitudes, illogical thought processes, neuroses, or psychotic tendencies.

Emotional stress from within may also originate from a variety of sources: rational concern over illness, plight of self or those dear or important to self, or over day-to-day happenings, events, and situations; or irrational and exaggerated concern over similar events in which poor mental attitudes, illogical thought processes, neuroses, or psychotic tendencies play a major role. Emotional stress from without may originate from the environment itself, from persons in the environment, or from perceived or real failures in progression toward a goal.

Examples of emotional stress of environmental origin are fires, storms, or safety hazards; difficult superiors at work, or recalcitrant children; failure in progression toward a goal or a loss on an important investment; choice of a workmate to a new post above your own; and divorce, and so on. Emotional stress is by far the most difficult to deal with in our modern society, and by far the most common cause of tension and fatigue. Emotionally charged situations or events are innumerable. Again, you must keep in mind the complex and constant and dynamic interplay that goes on between physical, mental, and emotionally derived stress, both from within and without the subject. The concept shown in Figure 7 is of value.

INTERRELATIONSHIP OF FACTORS PRODUCING FATIGUE

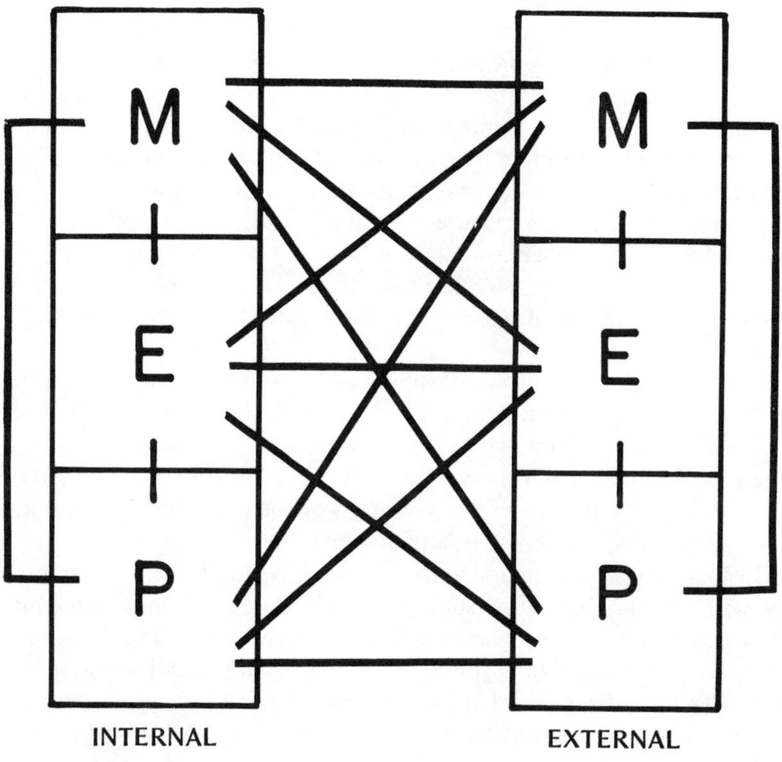

Mental = Mental E = Emotional P = Physical

Figure 7: Factors producing fatigue may be classified as mental (M), emotional (E), or physical (P).

These factors may arise from within the subject (internal) or from without (external, environmental). Such factors never operate independently, but are in constant, dynamic equilibrium with all other factors, as represented by the interconnecting lines shown above. As you have already seen, the relative size of each factor is subject to great variation from one to another segment of time.

Types of Stress (as to origin). A look at the Strife-Goal Concept discussed above reminds us that stress may originate from you, your environment, or from the goal(s) you are pursuing.

Recall that stress originating from within yourself may be due to such factors as inadequate personality, neuropsychiatric disorders (neuroses, psychoses, depression), physical disease or deprivation syndromes, inadequate training, unrealistic desires and philosophies, and so on. Some of these I have already considered. The more important ones are considered in greater depth in the next section.

As already pointed out, the environment in which you work and play may be either hostile or friendly, antagonistic or helpful, conducive to stress or conducive to serenity. Stress may arise from your environment as a result of physical surroundings (work, home, leisure); interpersonal relationships (home, work, leisure); or obstacles in the path to your goal.

Working in a pleasant atmosphere in which ideal conditions of temperature and humidity are maintained (if indoors) is much less likely to cause physical stress and illness than working under conditions where no such control prevails and there is exposure to extremes of heat and cold. Living in a comfortable home in an area where you have no concern over sanitary living conditions is likewise considerably less stressful than if living under conditions where prevention of disease is a constant problem (for example, in a mission field).

Interpersonal relationships at home, at work, or during leisure hours may likewise be sources of stress or of release from stress. The tired office worker who is habitually encountered by disruptive children when he gets home finds his home environment a source of stress. The bank clerk who aspires to reach new heights in the banking world is stressed by a superior vp whose personality clashes with hers at every turn.

Obstacles between you and your goal are a part of the environment, and they may take the form of persons, places, or things. The mountain climber finds a glacier an obstacle when it intervenes between him and the mountain peak lying just beyond. The young man aspiring to marry is stressed by his fiancee's father's disapproval of the marriage. The money necessary to make a promising investment may be an obstacle when it is lacking or insufficient.

Goals are so all-important as sources of chronic tension-fatigue that they are considered in a later chapter in even greater depth.

The Magnitude of Stress. Stress not only has quality (different types and origins), but quantity (magnitude). Magnitude is the product of intensity and duration, which is equivalent to saying that a pressure of, say five pounds per square inch for ten hours has the same effect as ten pounds per square inch for five hours. In other words the more intense the stress, the less time is required for it to exert a deleterious effect. On the other hand even stress of low degree, if continued sufficiently long, can have a telling effect on you. For example it has been clearly shown that control-tower workers in major airports develop stress diseases—hypertension, ulcers, cardiovascular dis-

THE SOCIAL READJUSTMENT RATING SCALE*

	Life Event	Mean Value
1.	Death of spouse	100
2.	Divorce	73
3.	Marital separation from mate	65
4.	Detention in jail or other institution	63
5.	Death of a close family member	63
6.	Major personal injury or illness	53
7.	Marriage	50
8.	Being fired at work	47
9.	Marital reconciliation with mate	45
10.	Retirement from work	45
11.	Major change in the health or behavior of a family member	44
12.	Pregnancy	40
13.	Sexual difficulties	39
14.	Gaining a new family member (through birth, adoption, oldster moving in, etc.)	39
15.	Major business readjustment (merger, reorganization, bankruptcy, etc.)	39
16.	Major change in financial state (a lot worse off or a lot better off than usual)	38
17.	Death of a close friend	37
18.	Changing to a different line of work	36
19.	Major change in the number of arguments with spouse (either a lot more or a lot less than usual regarding childrearing, personal habits, etc.)	35
20.	Taking on a mortgage greater than $10,000 (purchasing a home, business, etc.)	31
21.	Foreclosure on a mortgage or loan	30
22.	Major change in responsibilities at work (promotion, demotion, lateral transfer)	29
23.	Son or daughter leaving home (marriage, attending college, etc.)	29
24.	In-law troubles	29

* From T.H. Holmes and R.H. Rahe, "The Social Readjustment Rating Scale," *Journal of Psychosomatic Research,* 11 (1967): 213-218. Reprinted with permission of Thomas H. Holmes, M.D., Department of Psychiatry and Behavioral Sciences, University of Washington School of Medicine, Seattle, Washington 98195, and Pergamon Press Inc., Fairview Park, Elmsford, New York 10523.

Life Event	Mean Value
25. Outstanding personal achievement	28
26. Spouse beginning or ceasing work outside the home	26
27. Beginning or ceasing formal schooling	26
28. Major change in living conditions (building a new home, remodeling, deterioration of home or neighborhood)	25
29. Revision of personal habits (dress, manners, associations, etc.)	24
30. Troubles with the boss	23
31. Major change in working hours or conditions	20
32. Change in residence	20
33. Changing to a new school	20
34. Major change in usual type or amount of recreation	19
35. Major change in church activities (a lot more or a lot less than usual)	19
36. Major change in social activities (clubs, dancing, movies, visiting, etc.)	18
37. Taking on a mortgage or loan less than $10,000 (purchasing a car, television, freezer, etc.)	17
38. Major change in sleeping habits (a lot more or a lot less sleep, or change in part of day when asleep)	16
39. Major change in number of family get-togethers (a lot more or a lot less than usual)	15
40. Major change in eating habits (a lot more or a lot less food intake, or very different meal hours or surroundings)	15
41. Vacation	13
42. Christmas	12
43. Minor violations of the law (traffic tickets, jaywalking, disturbing the peace, etc.)	11

ease—at a much faster rate than persons engaged in similar activity in small airports. This is an example of the effect of intense stress exerted over a relatively short period of time. On the other hand, even control-tower workers in smaller airports may develop ulcers and high blood pressure if they continue long enough in their occupation.

Different life situations beget different degrees of stress. One such list is presented on the following pages. Note that the stress situations given the highest rating are the more intense, that is they give rise to the deeper and more violent emotions.

Total Stress. The total stress being exerted at any one time upon you is the sum total of all stresses acting upon you. It may be depicted somewhat as follows:

Job Stress + Family Stress + Financial Stress
+ Personal (Health) Problems = Total Stress

How any one individual handles his total stress depends upon personality structure and background (genetics), and training or education, among other things. A total stress of $2x$ may cause all sorts of anxiety reactions and psychosomatic disease in a friend with a brittle personality structure and poor training. If you have a solid personality and excellent training, it may cause hardly a ripple. On the other hand, if the order of total stress is raised to $10x$, it may cause even you to crumble. Some very excellent work in psychosomatic disease has indicated that there is no person alive who cannot, if subjected to sufficient stress, be made to manifest psychiatric or somatic symptoms.

Stress, then, is total environment working upon a given total individual. In the diagram below, environmental pressures (stress) are represented as acting upon a balloon (you). If your personality structure, background, training, and coping techniques are sufficiently strong to resist such pressures, you will not be "dangerously expanded" by your total stress. You may even become the stronger for any given experience. If such is not the case, you may "explode" when beset by the same set of circumstances (Figure 8).

The physiologic reaction to stress, which is tension, is proportionate to the degree of stress. In turn, emotional fatigue, which is a physiologic byproduct of tension, is proportional to the tension. It is extremely important that this concept be kept in mind.

Some Case Studies

Now let's look at some examples in the light of what you have learned. Jack is our subject. He is a sprinter whose goal is to run one hundred yards in the fastest possible time. Assuming that the track is fast and the wind and weather are favorable, his time will be determined largely by intrinsic factors such as his physical makeup, state of health, training and track experience, and desire to win (competitiveness). The goal is clearly defined and is presumably desirable to Jack, and there are no obstacles on the track. The environment is conducive physically, and if he has teammates present, the emotional aspects are doubtless a plus factor.

Ron is a 220 hurdler. He runs on the same day under the same conditions as Jack, but his point of departure and his finish line are farther apart, and there are numerous obstacles interposed between start and finish.

STRESS AND RESISTANCE TO STRESS

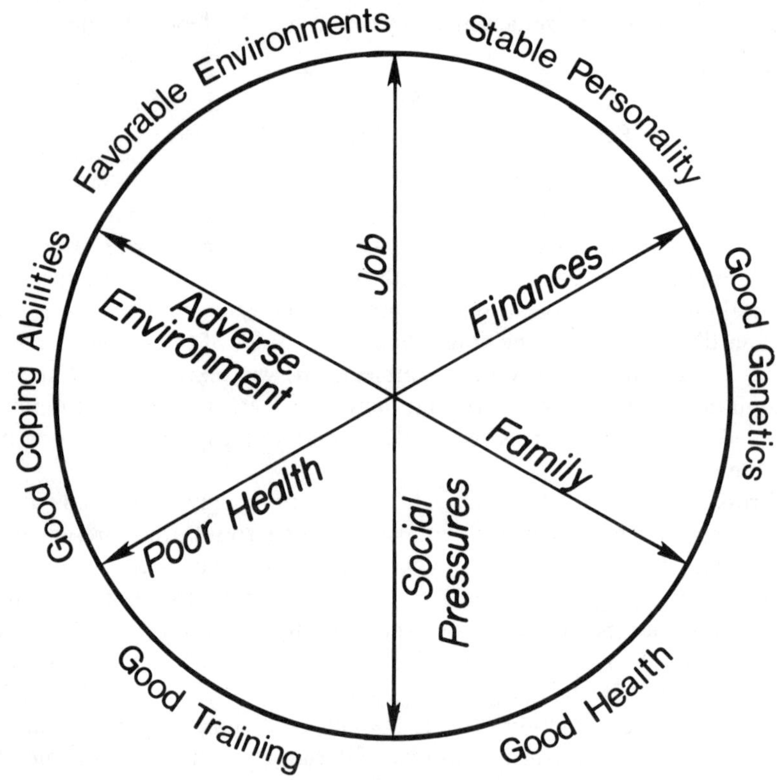

Figure 8: At any given moment, one or more stress factors (some of which are shown here inside the circle, or "balloon") may be operative in a given subject. These are countered by antistress factors such as those shown here on the oyter surface of the balloon. If stress is too great to be countered, the balloon expands to eventual rupture and collapse (exhaustion).

Since chronic stress begets chronic fatigue, the greater the ratio of stress to antistress factors, or the less able one is to cope with stress, the greater the resultant fatigue. Fatigue is directly proportional to the number and magnitude of all stress factors, and inversely proportional to the number and magnitude of all antistress factors, in operation at any given time.

Susan runs the marathon. Her goal is to traverse a prescribed twenty-six-mile path across country. Again, essentially the same factors come into play as with Jack, but Susan's goal is farther removed from the starting point and the terrain she must traverse more filled with obstacles. Assuming that she must run on a different day in wet weather, the environment has ganged up against her as well.

Should the intrinsic factors in the three runners be very nearly the same, the environment imposes greater stress on Ron than on Jack, and more on Susan than either of the other two. On the other hand, if Susan is a superbly trained, highly competitive "natural," her run may be less stressful to her than the runs of Jack or Ron are to them if they are poorly trained or have recently been ill (intrinsic factors).

Sam. Now let's get acquainted with Sam, our business executive who is typical of the complainant with the chronic-fatigue syndrome. On first examination he may appear to have little or nothing in common with our athletes, but on closer examination it becomes obvious that he has a great deal in common. There are also differences, and it is in these that the explanation of Sam's chronic fatigue lies.

Sam, at age fifty, runs his empire with a brace of telephones, a couple of assistants, and a cigarette perched precariously in the corner of his mouth. He is thirty pounds overweight, has high blood pressure, and his blood "fats" (cholesterol and triglycerides) are out of bounds. But you should see that house of his on Swank Hill, and that chauffered Caddy that he sports to and from his office. In another few years, Sam will be carried, feet first, to another Caddy—a long, black one—for his last ride, and everyone will keep on talking for a month or two about what he left behind. Sam had it made! And he had worked like the very devil for it! Eighteen, twenty hours a day. Never slept. Stayed late at the office or brought his work home with him. Coffee was his get-up and all-morning beverage, and cocktails his mainstay at noon and in the evening. He kept some downers on hand to help him get off to sleep when he couldn't unwind. Yes, Sam was a real Horatio Alger package of big, fat success. Well-trained. Shrewd as a fox. And always on the go—like a windmill in a hurricane. Sam had cut his teeth on the motto: be a winner or die trying. Well, he was a winner, and he was soon to die trying to hold on to his gains.

Sam and Our Runners. What do Sam and our track athletes have in common? Obviously each has a goal. Also each must strive to reach that goal. Each must contend with the environment and with certain obstacles to attain the goal. And each possesses certain intrinsic capabilities and shortcomings which affect the ease or difficulty with which the goal is attained.

But here the similarities end and the differences begin. First the goal. The goal of the track athlete is to win a race, a well-defined, clear-cut sort of thing. Sam's goal, on the other hand, is to succeed in life. Such success is a poorly defined, abstract goal, loaded with complexities, elusive, slippery, and often vague.

Next, the strife or stress. It differs in both quality and quantity. Qualitatively, the runners are striving primarily on a physical plane, while Sam is striving chiefly with mind and emotions. Quantitively, Jack strives for a few seconds, Ron a few seconds longer, and Susan for three and a half or four hours. On the other hand, Sam is in his fray hour after hour, day after day, week after week, year after year. In short, our runner friends' stress is *acute* and quickly resolved by vigorous physical activity, while Sam's is *chronic* and poorly resolved, if at all, by ill-defined measures haphazardly conceived. The runners must contend with their environment, albeit somewhat hostile to Susan, for only a brief segment of time. Sam must contend with his year after year in all its chameleonic aspects, at times hostile, at times friendly, but always demanding and inexorable and complex. The obstacles in the paths of the runners, although more formidable in the case of Susan and Ron than in that of Jack, are well-defined and forthrightly dealt with, whereas obstacles in the path of Sam are often elusive, intangible, and difficult to define.

In short, our runners fight a battle—quickly, decisively—for a clear-cut goal. Sam, on the other hand, fights a war, and to win he must fight many battles—long and drawn-out, often never decided—for an elusive and seemingly ever-retreating goal.

The Stress of Strife and a Way of Life

While the stress of strife is common both to the runners and to Sam, the stress of life, or of a way of life, is peculiar to Sam. Sam's way of life is the American way—the way of civilization and of success-oriented society, of competition and ambition, of industrialization and urbanization. To a primitive in Africa, success is food on the table and the shelter of a grass hut. But not to Sam. Sam and his several million counterparts around the globe have been indoctrinated in the concept that success, American style, is made up of a bank account, a couple of swank automobiles, and a house on Manor Hill—each of these possessions bigger and better than the Joneses. Also, Sam must be educated; and one degree won't do anymore. Moreover, he must raise his family in the grand style: expensive boats, trips abroad, the best schools for his kids. And to show for it all, Sam collects credit cards, mortgages, and a high tax bracket, all of which must be supported by our hero day after day, month after month, year after year.

Is it any wonder that Sam is up at daybreak, prying open his eyes with a potful of coffee and beginning his daily pack or two of cigarettes, mushing through the morning paper so he can talk intelligently about the mad, mad world? He eats a breakfast that would make a cardiologist cringe—a couple of eggs with side orders of buttered toast and ham. He shaves, showers, and downs a pep pill, then makes a mad dash for the bus. He disembarks in front of the office, elevators up to the tenth floor just a fringe ahead of the boss, and dives into a mountain of work which will never be finished but only frenziedly attacked from day to day.

He'll attend conferences, smoke more cigarettes, drink more coffee, yak on the telephone, and sit, sit, sit. He'll sit for the conferences, for the coffee-break, for the cigarettes, for the high-fat lunch and, after an afternoon of more of the same, he'll pack his briefcase and head for home, where he'll sit and have a martini or two and a cigarette before trouncing on that well-marbled steak with creamed potato, preceded by a salad with cream-cheese dressing, and followed by a chunk of Black Forest cake washed down with more coffee and topped off with a cigarette. Then, after a brief set-to with bad news on the TV, it's sit and work, later a midnight raid on the ice cream and cake, and at length a downer and to bed for a quick five in the land of restless Nod.

Then the alarm. And the rat race is on again. Day after day after endless day. For what? To succeed! To manufacture a private world out of long, pressure-packed hours fueled with fatty meat, butter, and eggs, washed down with coffee and alcohol, and fumigated with tobacco smoke—all from the seat of the pants. Yes, success is adding pounds to the waist for the sake of putting pounds in the bank. It's watching the credit rating climb along with the blood pressure. It's matching fat bankrolls with fat diets. It's playing Russian roulette for the most expensive piece of property you'll ever own—a plot in the cemetery. That's success, American style. And Sam, at fifty-two, collected a $10,000 headstone to prove it.

Operating as they do under the chronic stress of multiple stressor agents, shooting for a goal as ill-defined as chronic success in an environment that is chronically demanding, it is little wonder that the Sams of this world are chronically tense and chronically tired.

Chronic Tension = Chronic Fatigue

Sam is chronically preparing for fight or flight. His adrenal glands are being repetitively stimulated by numerous stimuli—intrinsic, environmental, and goal oriented. Time after time he must meet a challenge with subtle, but definite increases in blood pressure and pulse rate and muscle tension, differing only in degree from the increases that appear just before and during the running of a race.

Over the long haul, Sam adapts to repeated stimuli, as in the G.A.S. of Selye, but with the passage of years, his resistance begins to falter. The repeated outpourings of adrenalin and adrenal corticoids eventually lead to a chronic overreaction, the result of which is chronic, unrelenting tension.

And *chronic tension means chronic fatigue*! Why? Look at Figure 5 again. Note that the precise purpose of tension buildup is to enable the organism to fight or flee, the natural aftermath of which is fatigue. In other words, after a man fights, he is tired. After a man runs, he is tired. Fatigue is the natural end product of released tension. But what if a man prepares to run, or to fight, but never quite gets around to the actual action? Tension builds up, but is never fully released. It is instead recycled again and again (Figure 9). Tension remains unreleased, in the case of Sam, over protracted periods of time. It is as though Sam were perpetually under the starter's gun, but the physical release of muscles in action never comes as it does for our

THE TENSION CYCLE IN MODERN CIVILIZATION

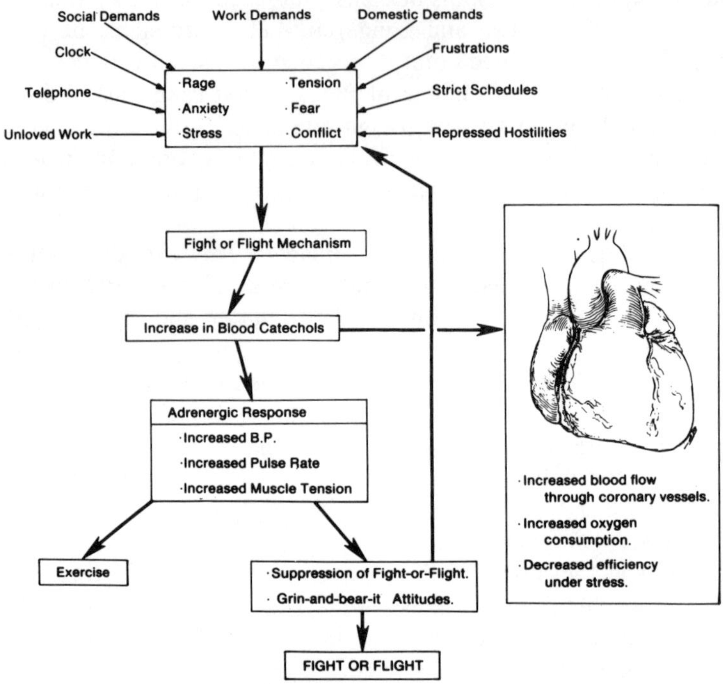

*Figure 9:** Physiologically, modern man responds to the tensions of modern living much as he does to danger. The same fight-or-flight mechanism is set in motion repeatedly, with a damaging, chronically recurrent elevation in blood catechols (adrenalin and noradrenalin) leading to a chronically recurring adrenergic response (Figure 5). But in modern fight or flight, the natural skeletal muscle outlet for these tensions is blocked by suppressions, repressions, and grin-and-bear-it attitudes. The result is a cycle of still more stress – and chronic fatigue. Exercise is the perfect substitute for fight or flight, a readily available and natural means of breaking the cycle.

runner friends. So after a period of adaptation, chronic fatigue sets in, partly because of the cumulative effect of the physiologic by-products of tension, but largely because the mind apparently interprets unreleased tension in terms of fatigue. Sam may sleep poorly, for example, because the event for which he tensed has never come off. True, the stress imposed upon Sam is primarily mental, or emotional, in nature. But the tension it begets requires for ultimate release the self-same action of muscle and sinew that releases the tension of the track athletes—action that never comes.

Let's follow the evolution of Sam from his early ancestry, and the reason for this becomes more apparent.

* From M.F. Graham, M.D., *Prescription for Life,* (New York: McKay, 1966). Reprinted with permission.

The Evolution of Tension—A Timely Tale

Let's go back a long, long way to the time when all that Sam's ancestors owned were a cave and a club. What was success then? Money in the bank? A closet full of $200 suits? A private airplane? No, success was fresh, raw meat on the floor; a cave with a view; coming in first in a race with a dinosaur. It was 98 percent muscle, 2 percent brain. Tomorrow would take care of itself. There was enough of today to make a man sleep from sheer exhaustion. The only insurance was a good set of legs and a strong pair of arms.

But one day between fang-fests a man sat lazily clinking a set of flints together—a stone ax against a spearhead—and sparks flew into a nearby clump of dead grass. A flame sprung, and fire was born. And thereafter man cooked his kill and shaped more perfectly the rock in the flame, and kept the wild beast at bay. There were better spears and better arrows, there was more meat on the floor and better protection against the dangers that lurked in the night. And a little less—just a little less—need for good legs.

Then man banded together around the fire and learned of strength in numbers, the circling of the kill, the multiplied force of many. And tribes were born and work divided. And with it came a little less—just a little less—need for legs.

Then one day, with his ax, a man lazily hacked a furrow in the ground and, accidentally, flipped a seed or two from a wild gourd he was eating at the fallow soil. He forgot it for a time, and then he saw, early in a morning mist, a tiny burst of green, two, three, wherever a seed had fallen. And farming was born—the predetermined, deliberate working of the soil for food. And with it man ceased, in part, his nomadic wanderings in quest of meat and settled green valleys where corn would come in season and food could be stored with anticipation rather than tracked in desperation. Farming built villages, and man was safer from his environment, safer from starvation, more secure. But the planting of corn could not match in muscular effort the eternal quest for the kill. So, but a little, man's needs for his legs dwindled ever so slightly.

And over the years came, in rapid successions as centuries go, the harnessing of beasts and the discovery of the wheel. And man commanded that beast do his work. And the wheel came slowly between man's feet and the good earth. And man came to depend less and less and less on his legs.

Then came iron! And stone was suddenly outmoded. The stone-axed man was no match for his ironclad antagonist. And the beasts that lurked in the shadows were pushed ever farther away from the tribal fire of the village. Serendipity had placed a premium on that part of man that lay between his ears—his brain. With it he could conquer all. With it there was, strangely, less and less need to run.

And then, as the pages of a book flip wildly in a rising wind, there came in close succession gunpowder, steam, electricity, machinery, and finally, the contraption that broke man's legs in two, the automobile. And all the while man's first enemy, the wild beast, receded farther and farther into the shadows of history, and in its place arose man's worst enemy (physiologically speaking)—man himself. He began to communicate with long wires, then with invisible waves. He traveled first with the speed of his legs, but in due time with the speed of sound. And finally came the bomb! Power undreamed of. Destructiveness unparalleled. Future unlimited. Electronic marvelry. Rocketry. Man looking for new worlds to conquer. Man racing for the moon.

And man sitting on his big, fat can! Drinking up TV by the hour. And on the job, pushing buttons, pulling levers, pushing a pencil. The farm? Grandpa stuff. The city's the life. Bright lights, soft living. And money. And the race is on, but now run not with the legs, but with the brain. The race for the biggest house with the biggest garage with the biggest car and the best TV set on the block. Legs? They still come in handy now and then. Like getting to and from the nearest automobile. Or to the nearest elevator. Or from the dinner table to the TV set. But for walking? For running? For keeping old sabertooth from the door? For literally bringing home the bacon? How crude, how ancient, can you get? This is a refined age. We pick our teeth now with gold toothpicks, not fish ribs. We fill our larders by our wits, not our spears. What counts is what you can count in thousands, millions, even billions. And the dollar sign is the sign of the times!

Indeed, man has come a long, long way. From cave to penthouse. Stone ax to H-bomb. Unikill to megakill. Sugar cane to cane sugar. Fence row to skid row. Sand between the toes to fancy hose. He's been refined, wined, and dined on easy living. He can point to the Sams of the world and say he's arrived. And those that aren't there yet, individuals or nations, aren't about to quit until they get there! Until they get their share of the brass rings and the muckety-muck.

But do you know what? Sam has outdone himself. In running off and leaving his legs, he's made a bum swap, a poor trade. He's been suckered into quicksand and, most of the time, is blissfully unaware of it. Not that atomic power doesn't have mule power beat by a few thousand megatons. Or that foam rubber doesn't make a heck of a lot softer bed than a cave floor. Or that tractors can't plow ten furrows far, far straighter and faster than a burro can just one. Or that autos and airplanes haven't made the world a lot smaller and closer-knit than oxcarts. Not at all. What is meant is that man has socially and industrially and technically evolved so rapidly that his mind has left his body somewhere in the peatbogs of the past. For man's physiologic machinery remains the same as it was when all that stood between him and that charging mammoth was his little ol' ax and a good pair of legs. And those adrenals react to danger in the same old way. But as he has traded caves for castles, clubs for guns, tiger skins for sheep skins, he has also traded the tension of mortal combat—resolved the minute it was born by fight or flight—for the tension of keeping up with the Joneses, a tension all too often never resolved at all. He could fight a dino to the death; in fact, he had to then and there.

But Sam dare not fight the boss! Even though Sam is spoiling for a fight, even though that promotion should have been his! Even though he's worked so very long, so very hard. Even though his kids deserve as much as the Jones kids, the same chances, the same livery, the same good life. But with the bills piling up and the upkeep of the new house climbing, Sam can't afford a fight. So the modern Sam clinches his fists and swallows his pride and stews inside. His pulse races and his blood pressure climbs and his blood "fats" soar; and they keep on racing and climbing and soaring, day after day, month after month, year after year. For on the merry-go-round of success, if it's not the boss it's someone else; if it's not the job it's something else. So keep plugging, and the racing pulse and the climbing pressure and the soaring fat be damned. True, Sam's ancestors' pulses and pressures and fats also increased when faced with danger—it's basic preparation for fight or flight—but they found quick release. They did not simmer and fume, fanned with the anxieties and frustrations and repressed hostilities of months and years, and in so doing kill the hunter instead of the prey.

If by involution is meant, as Webster says, becoming involved, man's social evolution has led to his hopeless involution. Man is involved, intricately, hopelessly, with his environment. He has traded clearly discernible dangers without for ill-defined fears and threats within and, like a spider spinning a web, he has become hopelessly entangled therein himself. He has traded physical toughness, physical fitness if you will, for mental mania; that 80 percent of his body which is musculoskeletal for that 2 percent of him which is brain.

And who would belittle the trade had it not been made in toto, had fitness not been completely sacrificed on the altar of mentality? None would deny that an ounce of gray matter is worth a pound of muscle, whether in the dawn of human time or in the sun-dimming glare of a mushroom cloud. And who would argue that, whether manning a cannon or a cyclotron, mind is still, as always, the master of matter? Or who could be so fatuous as to contend that the mecca of mentality in which man finds himself striving for mastery is a totally bad, or unfortunate, state of affairs? This is not the point. The point is that, paradoxically, man's mind has run away from his legs. His brain has mapped inerrantly, albeit sometimes circuitously, the long, laborious pathway from the sunrise to the noonday of human achievement, but in the process it forgot that man was, physiologically, born to run—literally and figuratively—with his legs!

The conquest of four-footed dangers without was indeed a milestone of progress, a feat of mentality, only one of many that sets man apart from the beasts he conquered. But with the steady subjugation and rearrangement of his physical environment over the centuries man has disarranged and sadly neglected his internal milieu. Sam's early ancestors had puny minds and powerful bodies. Sam, by virtue of the rearrangement of his environment, had just the opposite—a powerful mind housed in a prematurely tired and degenerated body. Thus it becomes a fair question: can either combination lead man to his ultimate destiny? Indeed not! Sam's first ancestor was no more complete a man than is Sam himself. In fact, both were and are woefully incomplete, inadequate representatives of the whole man. Both were and are, at either end of the scale, but half a man. For the whole man is sound mind in sound body, and I might add, sound spirit.

The more affluent a society the more complex must become the machinery by which it perpetuates itself. Complexity breeds complexity. Pressures breed pressures. And it is an unfortunate and deadly paradox that complexity has neither time nor inclination nor stomach for simplicity. Fishcakes and rice, a good diet to aid in prevention of heart attacks, may be fine fare for backward simpletons, but only marbled steaks and creamed dressings belong on fine uptown china. Running may be a very necessary part of making a rickshaw go, a backward custom for a backward people, but it's downright stupid to huff and puff to work on a bicycle when but a smidgeon of pressure on an accelerator will do the same job in a third the time.

The Sams of the world are blind. They cannot see simply because they do not have time to see. They equate success with complexity, and complexity—involvement—demands their full attention. There is no time for simplicity. If one is to reach the pinnacle of success he must hurry. And to hurry means to move, quickly, efficiently; there is simply no place for legs when wheels and levers and buttons work their magic so quickly. The old has given way to the new. This is progress? This is civilization, a complex, stressful, intricate, demanding hodge-podge of servile halfmen, of hurried and harried, tense and tired, bulging, belt-lined, shiny-seated Sams.

Contrast Sam's world with that of a peaceful village high in the Andes, a village known as Vilcabamba. World-renowned for the health and longevity of its residents, it boasts a population of 819, with seven men and two women over the century mark. A paltry few, you say. But if the United States did as well it would count 2,500,000 centenarians instead of its fewer than 7,000. What's more the villagers of this quiet little community don't seem to get sick. They hear well, see well, and remain mentally alert and physically active well into their nineties and beyond. They are a simple and dignified people that subsist on natural foods, walk a great deal, and work hard, chiefly outdoors.

Isolated from the stresses of Sam's civilized world, their low-caloric, chiefly starch diet would drive a modern nutritionist up the wall.

There are accurate reports of Sams, badly crippled with heart disease, who after spending months in the village have come away new men.

What's the lesson? That premature illness and death, diseases of adaptation, and emotional disorders are products of complex living, with its chronic tension and its chronic fatigue. The villagers of Vilcabamba will never drive a Cadillac or own a home on Swank Hill. And their simple fare will be earned by the sweat of their brow. But Sam will never see one half—or maybe one third—of their sunsets. And most of the ones he sees he'll be too tired to enjoy.

Iatrogenic Fatigue

As previously stated the term *iatrogenic* means "physician-induced." When the patient medicates or otherwise prescribes for himself, such a term, in its broadest interpretation, would of necessity mean patient-induced also. Prescriptions may utilize a variety of modalities: drugs, physical measures, rest and recreations, environmental manipulation, and so on. In terms of fatigue production, drugs undoubtedly head the list.

Drugs

Ours is a drug culture, as evidenced by reams of data. For instance, more than 75 million Americans consume at least one drug a week, most of them every day. $2.6 billion a year is spent on off-the-shelf medications and another $11 billion a year on prescription drugs in the United States. Based on a report by the United States Census Bureau for 1974, the following breakdown on drug consumption is most revealing:

*1974 U.S. Drug Consumption in Millions of Dollars at Manufacturers Selling Price.**

Systemic (taken internally) antibiotics	783
Tranquilizers and other psychotherapeutic agents	590
Aspirin combinations	224
Other internal analgesics (pain-killers) and antipyretics (antifever)	204
Salicylates (including aspirin)	110
Antidepressants	81
Appetite suppressants (excluding amphetamine)	44
Amphetamines	21
Barbiturates	21

*To reflect consumption at consumer prices, multiply these figures by two.

Grouping the above on a functional basis, it is obvious that aside from antibiotic consumption (most of it ineffective and inappropriately used, such as penicillin for the common cold), the tranquilizer group heads the list ($590), followed closely by aspirin or aspirin-related compounds ($538). This means that in 1974 the average person in the United States spent about seven dollars for systemic antibiotics, six dollars for psychotherapeutic agents, and five dollars for nonnarcotic analgesics such as aspirin. What could speak more eloquently of the headache and fatigue-besetting tensions that buffet the average citizen of the good ol' US of A?

And our consumption of such drugs leaps upward annually. For example, the sale of over-the-counter analgesics (such as aspirins) increased by $17.8 million (5.2 percent) over the preceding year, and that of prescribed analgesics by $32.3 million (12.5 percent).* Our complex society steadily grows more and more complex, and as it does so, the use of tension-relieving drugs grows with it. One could utilize the consumption of such drugs as an index of the overall stressfullness of the social climate generated by a given way of life. It is interesting, in this regard, that the consumption of such drugs in Great Britain (a country with a similar social structure) closely parallels that in the United States.

Drug utilization begins early in stressful cultures. One survey has indicated that on any given day in a certain county in New York, one child in three (and one mother in two) is taking some medication (predominantly vitamins, aspirin, and cold remedies). Taking medication, a practice begun at an early age, may be more American than apple pie.

Such statistics do not indicate the even greater usage of such drugs as alcohol and tobacco, which are considered in some detail shortly.

Sedatives. "Beginning in the teen years and persisting through the lean years," downers are gulped by the bushels in this country. Conservative estimates have it that 25 to 50 percent of all Americans over forty use hypnotics or tranquilizers. Sedative-hypnotics are prescribed more than any group of medications in the world (128 million prescriptions in the United States in 1976).

The common misconception, even among most physicians, is that such drugs are short-enough acting that they leave no hangover effect the following day. This is far from the truth. No sedative (indeed, no drug!) exists—barbiturate, soporific, or otherwise—which is entirely free of side-effects. Sedatives are all capable of producing day-after somnolence, lethargy, even depression, the feeling of fatigue.

Moreover, sedatives eventually impair sleep, inasmuch as the user practically always develops tolerance and dependency. With only one or two exceptions, all sleeping pills cause insomnia or worsen it. Total sleep time may increase at first, but within a week or two it declines, sometimes to a level below that before medication was begun. Increase in the dose causes repetition of the cycle, and the larger the dose the more dependent the patient. He may become tolerant of tremendous doses of the drug within a few months, yet still suffer from insomnia. Withdrawal of the drug produces total sleeplessness or very disturbed sleep.

Similar dependency can result with any other compound to which rapid tolerance develops, including alcohol (the chronic ingestion of which leads to insomnia) and over-the-counter sleep drugs. It is, in fact, the opinion of many sleep experts that such over-the-counter drugs should not be sold since such compounds are ordinarily misused and create new problems rather than solve old ones.

The common approach is downers at night and uppers in the morning, with the user not realizing that uppers may themselves have fatigue-

*Based on FDC reports.

producing effects which, in conjunction with increasingly severe hangovers from sedatives, simply amplify the production of fatigue. Even coffee, as we shall see, is capable of producing all sorts of severe problems related to fatigue.

Tranquilizers. In their eternal quest for tranquility in an anything-but-tranquil society, Americans lean on tranquilizers like cripples lean on crutches. While such drugs do have an ameliorating effect on tension and anxiety, habitual usage all too often produces side effects which, like sedatives, may be worse, or as bad as, the problem for which they are taken. All too often in taking tranquilizers, one simply trades one problem for another—in this instance, anxiety or tension for fatigue. As is obvious from even a cursory perusal of the subject in the PDR,* drowsiness and fatigue are among the more frequently encountered side effects of most tranquilizers in common use today. Other possible adverse effects include confusion, depression, headache, insomnia, and sleep disturbances, none of which are calculated to help the problem of chronic fatigue.

It is safe to say that the fatigued individual who uses tranquilizers with any degree of regularity is compounding his problem considerably, often greatly. In fact, it is impossible to manage chronic fatigue successfully if the indiscriminate use of tranquilizers is practiced. It's a great deal like strapping another pack on an already-tired mountain climber.

Analgesics. Chief of the analgesics (pain-relievers) is everyone's old standby, aspirin. The daily intake of aspirin by Americans is estimated at 46.5 tons (nearly 140 million tablets). The hub of every medicine cabinet, it has been used in the treatment of every ache and pain known to man. Administered by physician and layman alike, "take an aspirin" has become the emergency treatment for every ailment.

While aspirin, by and large, is a relatively safe drug (it would have to be to survive the usage to which it has been put), it is capable of producing some severe side effects, effects which are relatively unknown to laymen and too poorly known by most physicians.

The most severe of these side effects is an entity known as "salicylism," characterized by headache, dizziness, ringing in the ears, and fatigue. Some persons exhibit a sensitivity reaction to aspirin which can produce fatigue as an adjunctive finding.

Aspirin is a good example of a drug used so widely and with such a blase attitude that little thought is given to the adverse effects it is capable of producing. It underscores the old aphorism in medicine, "There is no never and no always," which is to say that there is no such thing as a drug without the potential for doing harm, often more harm than good.

Antibiotics. Since Alexander Fleming's discovery of penicillin, microbes have been dealt a severe blow by a veritable avalanche of antibiotics, all with potentially serious adverse effects, some more so than others. Much atten-

**Physicians Desk Reference* (Oradell, N.J.: Medical Economics Co., 1976).

tion has been directed to the allergic manifestations of such drugs—rashes, joint problems, even death-dealing anaphylaxis—but the more subtle adverse effects, among which is fatigue, are seldom called to mind.

There is no antibiotic or chemotherapeutic agent (such as sulfa) which is not capable of causing fatigue. If you thumb through the Physicians Desk Reference and contemplate the adverse reactions ascribed to different germ-killing agents, you will be astounded at the frequency with which fatigue appears and reappears as a potential side effect. The mechanism of fatigue-production by this group of drugs may relate to involvement of practically any body system—hematopoietic (blood-formation), central nervous system, liver, kidney.

When one considers that a high percentage of patients take unprescribed antibiotics (39 percent in one series), the potential problem becomes at once obvious. Medicinally classified drugs, of the type previously considered, are so numerous that to even attempt to allude to all of them would be a ponderous undertaking. Suffice it to say that any drug in any category presents the potential of producing an ill effect as well as, or rather than, a beneficial one. Hence in the consideration of a chronic fatigue problem you need always to call to mind any and every drug you might be ingesting with some regularity.

"Undrugs"

In this group are briefly considered drugs that are not ordinarily thought of as such, but which, nonetheless, possess all the potential hazards possessed by medicinally classified drugs.

Vitamins. If aspirin is taken for what ails you, then vitamins are taken just as freely for what doesn't ail you. Riding on a crest of alleged benefits ranging from the prevention of old age to the restoration of youth, the vitamin craze has made such an impact on the American populace that it is difficult to find a patient with any sort of ailment who has not given vitamins a whirl at effecting a cure.

1. The B bunch. Vitamin B-complex is constituted of B_1 (thiamin), B_2 (riboflavin), B_6 (pyridoxine), B_{12} (cyanocobalamin), nicotinamide, pantothenic acid, and lesser known constituents such as inositol and choline. By and large overdosage with these vitamins is difficult from the standpoint of causing adverse symptoms. Nicotinic acid or nicotinamide may cause dilatation of the peripheral blood vessels with transient flushing and headache, and sometimes fatigue, but large doses, unlikely to be encountered under ordinary circumstances, are required.

2. Vitamins A and D. These vitamins are capable of producing severe organ damage, especially to the kidneys and quite possibly to the arteries, when ingested in large quantities, and should never be taken medicinally unless expressly prescribed by a physician. Fatigue is only one of many symptoms which can result. The margin of safety with vitamin D is quite narrow, the toxic dose being only five to ten times the amount necessary to prevent serious bone disorders.

3. Vitamin C (ascorbic acid). While this vitamin appears to be relatively nontoxic, even in huge quantities, there is much that remains to be determined about the long-term effects of megadosage. Some studies now indicate that massive doses of this vitamin could be hazardous. In particular, aged preparations of vitamin C should not be used indiscreetly, inasmuch as degradation of the vitamin may occur with aging, with adverse effects on the urinary tract in particular.

4. Vitamin E. Most medical authorities agree that the only thing vitamin E lacks is a good indication for its use. Its name alone (tocopherol, which means the oil of fertility) has so tickled the public fancy that it ranks close to vitamin C as a prevent-all, this despite the fact that its ubiquity in nature renders the possibility of deficiency quite remote.

Being hawked and used nowadays for such entities as impotency, high blood pressure, and fatigue, this vitamin, in large doses, is known to cause fatigue in some individuals. The medical literature refers to cases in which persons taking vitamin E for some unrelated reason developed extreme fatigue, which disappeared when the vitamin E was stopped and which reappeared when given again on a trial basis. While there are numerous attestations to its use to fight fatigue, it must be recognized that in any given instance this vitamin may cause fatigue rather than relieve it.

Tobacco. Nicotine, one of the active ingredients of tobacco, is a central nervous system stimulant which can, in large doses, cause convulsions. In the doses encountered in cigarettes and cigars, it causes a release of adrenalin from the adrenal gland, with resultant rises in blood pressure and heart rate—in other words it has a stressor effect. As you have seen—and shall see further—the ultimate aftermath of stress is fatigue, whatever the stressor may be. Thus the habitual smoker is, insofar as his adrenals are concerned, participating in a series of short sprints which, when all added together, can impose a sizable fatigue effect. Hence the smoker who lights up to fight off that fatigue feeling is in reality "whipping a tired horse."

Not only do cigarettes produce fatigue through their nicotine effect, but they cause an increase in carboxyhemoglobin in the blood (a good measure of absorption of tobacco smoke). This compound is formed of carbon monoxide, a deadly poison, and the oxygen-carrying component of the blood, hemoglobin. The accumulation of this compound results in a lower concentration of oxyhemoglobin, a combination of oxygen with hemoglobin, so that the overall oxygen-carrying capacity of the blood is lowered. It is probably this effect that has long caused athletic coaches to realize that good athletes don't smoke; and good athletes to realize that they can become better ones by kicking the habit. Some authorities feel that because of the slower reflexes resulting from the effect of carboxyhemoglobin, smoking should be refrained from by airline pilots for at least six hours before flying.

Fatigue is a common complaint of the habitual smoker. It should be noted further that there is some evidence that certain personality types—the tense, anxious variety—are more likely to be cigarette-smokers; and that smoking is thus but one external symptom of internal tension. If this be so, then it is even more urgent that the tired smoker dispense with his senseless, costly habit.

Alcohol (Ethanol). Folklore and tradition cloud the issue of alcohol. Once thought to be a remedy for practically anything, whisky (*usquebaugh* in Gaelic for "water of life") was not so-named for nothing. Apparently most Americans take its root meaning (water of life) seriously. Of the 116.5 million over eighteen years of age, only 20 percent are abstainers. 110 percent drink sparingly, 30 percent moderately, 23.5 percent heavily, 10.6 percent are dependent drinkers, and 5.9 percent are slaves.

The acute effects of alcohol intoxication are generally well known—the morning-after headache, the gastrointestinal upset, the blahs and the fatigue. But the chronic effects of long-term alcohol usage in social amounts—one or two cocktails an evening—are not. What is coming to the light these days, more and more, is the ill-effects of such small-dose usage on heart, liver, and brain. There is accumulating evidence that heart muscle may undergo a peculiar sort of degeneration in regular alcohol users, even though they do not imbibe to the point of intoxication. It has been estimated that brain cells succumb to alcohol to the tune of several million per jigger. And fatty degeneration of the liver, long recognized in chronic alcoholics, is now thought to occur in more subtle form in the social drinker. Any or all of these organ effects may cause chronic fatigue.

Alcohol is not a food. It cannot supply building-blocks for tissue. Furthermore, it is habituating, and the occasional user commonly becomes the chronic user, with insomnia, improper eating habits, and vitamin deficiencies following. Tolerance results from the repeated use of alcohol, so that ever larger doses must be taken to procure the desired effect. Thus in a subtle manner fatigue may be introduced from a dietary standpoint.

Pharmacologists agree that, contrary to popular opinion, alcohol, rather than being a stimulant, is a primary depressant of the nervous system. In this respect it is as much an anesthetic as ether and chloroform. Its alleged stimulatory effect stems from its depression of inhibitory centers in the brain. The chronic user of alcohol, even in small doses, is subjecting himself to central-nervous-system depression, albeit to token extents. And depression is the handmaiden of fatigue. Hence the element of depression, whether as a cause or as an effect of alcohol usage, must come into consideration.

The chronic user of alcohol—the social drinker—will usually point out that a "little alcohol is good for digestion," or that a drink or two is "relaxing." Certain breakdown products of alcohol do have properties akin to morphine. If one equates fatigue with relaxation, then to a degree this may be true. But when I encounter such a person I always think of the fellow who stopped to talk to me one day as he was doing a ten-mile jaunt around a lake. Once a smoker and an inveterate social drinker, he is now a marathon runner. Giving up the cigarettes came relatively easy in the early course of his conditioning. But it wasn't until he quit the daily cocktails that he became a marathon runner. No one could ever convince him—or hundreds of others like him—that alcohol usage does not produce fatigue.

Coffee, Tea, and Cocoa. Some two and a half billion pounds of coffee are used in the United States each year—2.2 cups per day for the average consumer. And 60 to 65 percent of the 5.7 billion gallons of carbonated drinks consumed each year contain a caffeine additive. Such commonly used drinks contain caffeine or caffeine-related compounds which all possess the common property of stimulation of the central nervous system. And stimulation is followed by fatigue. Caffeine or caffeine-equivalent content of commonly used beverages of this type are as follows:

	per five-ounce cup
Regular percolator coffee	83 milligrams
Instant coffee	59 milligrams
Tea from bags	42 to 100 milligrams
Leaf tea	30 to 75 milligrams
Instant tea	30 to 60 milligrams
Cocoa or hot chocolate	50 milligrams
	per eight-ounce can
Cola drinks	30 milligrams
Small chocolate bars	25 milligrams average

The heavier a person is, the more caffeine he can tolerate without ill effect. And vice versa. For example, a sixty-pound child ingesting three cola drinks a day would derive the same net effect as a 175-pound man drinking eight cups of coffee a day. It is now being recognized more and more that anxiety, fatigue, and even neurotic tendencies are in large numbers of cases due solely to improper usage of such common drinks and foods. More is said of this later.

Capsule Summary

Americans do indeed exist in a drug culture. But the worst of it may be that they do so without knowledge or understanding of either its magnitude or its effects. If you are suffering from chronic fatigue and are to understand or to cope with your problem, it is mandatory that you come to grips with the drugs you ingest, whether they be prescribed or obtained over the counter or from a grocery shelf. Until you see coffee, alcohol, sedatives—whatever—in the light of their effect on your total well-being, your efforts to conquer the fatigue problem will be in vain.

CHAPTER 4

Recognition of Fatigue Types: What Kind of Fatigue?

Inasmuch as most cases of chronic fatigue are of emotional origin, that is they arise from chronic tension, cures per se are relatively rare. While cures are theoretically possible, so inextricably are most individuals involved with their environments and their life-styles, it is highly unlikely that such cures will be realized. Radical surgery would be required, and the patient is too often unwilling to undergo the surgery. This becomes more apparent as you go along through this chapter. Hence the word *management.* If you cannot relieve the problem entirely, there is much that can be done to ameliorate the condition. It is a great deal like treating a cancer. Many cases can be cured if the surgery is early enough and radical enough, but when, for one or another reason, it is not, one then turns to palliative procedures—in other words management designed to make life livable for the patient. Hence, whether you effect a cure or simply convert an intolerable into a tolerable situation depends to a large extent on the individual involved and on the environmental and goal complex in which you are bound.

For the sake of discussion, I first consider management of chronic fatigue from the standpoint of its chief content, that is whether it is chiefly physical, chiefly mental, or chiefly emotional. Such a differential diagnosis is not always easy. Seldom does chronic fatigue originate from a purely physical, purely mental, or purely emotional cause. There is, in fact, such an intertwining of the three spheres that it is often difficult to determine where the primary cause lies (see Figure 2). Nevertheless, an effort should be made in each instance to make such a determination, for the management of one type may vary greatly from that of another.

Physical Fatigue

Physical fatigue due to *organic disease* must always be ruled out first, and you should never be content, simply because the odds are four to one against chronic fatigue's arising from such disease, to play the odds and assume that your own case is not in this minority group. A careful physical examination by a competent physician is a sine qua non point of departure for the management of chronic fatigue.

What are some of the hallmarks of organic disease that should alert one to the likelihood that a medical problem exists as a cause of fatigue?

1. Fatigue growing perceptibly worse from week to week, when other factors in the life-style remain essentially unchanged.

2. Certain symptoms or signs of possible cancer—unexplained bleeding from a body orifice; change in bowel habits; change in appearance or size of a mole; presence of a mass, as in a breast or under the skin.

3. Enlargement of "kernels" in the neck or elsewhere.

4. Persistent headache, especially if worsening in frequency or severity and unrelieved by aspirin.

5. Persistently waning appetite.

6. Fever of any degree persisting over a period of days to weeks.

7. Persistent vomiting.

8. Persistent diarrhea.

9. Persistent pain anywhere in the body, even though the pain may be more nagging than excruciating.

10. Chronic cough, especially if productive of pus or blood.

11. Excessive thirst or hunger, especially if attended by excessive urination.

12. Breathlessness on mild exertion, especially if worsening perceptibly from day to day or week to week.

13. Episodes of rapid heartbeat, especially if abrupt and not precipitated by exercise; or irregular heartbeat ("extra" beats, "skipped" beats, etc.)

14. Recurrent dizziness.

15. Progressive weakness in performance of simple physical tasks.

16. Noticeable change in skin color (pallor, yellowness) or texture; or a persistent rash of any type; or relatively rapid loss of hair or change in nail texture.

17. Joint swelling or stiffness unrelated to injury or change in habit patterns.

18. Urinary frequency or discomfort.

19. Disturbances in hearing (deafness, ringing in ears).

20. Disturbances in vision (spots before eyes, double vision, rapidly developing changes in visual acuity).

The above by no means run the gamut of hints as to organic disease, and by the same token many of the above may be due to nonorganic causes. But a person who has experienced any of the foregoing in association with fatigue (or, for that matter, without) should see his physician as soon as possible.

Physical fatigue of *physiologic origin* can usually be diagnosed by the R and R test, rest and refueling. Physiologic fatigue represents an imbalance between physical energy output and the restorative influence of rest and refueling. Thus if fatigue be principally of physiologic origin, the complainer usually presents the following picture:

1. He possesses no significant symptoms or signs suggestive of organic disease (as listed in the preceding symptoms).

2. Careful questioning usually makes it evident that the energy requirements for a day's work are disproportionately excessive for the time available for recuperation. For example: John was a seventeen-year-old high school student whose only complaint was fatigue which began, incidentally, shortly after the beginning of the school term. Questioning revealed that the boy worked in a filling station from after school to midnight and all day on Saturday and Sunday. He sometimes studied until two A.M. after he got off work during the week, and Saturday nights were for dating. He averaged no more than five hours sleep a night. It is not difficult for anyone to establish the cause—and the cure—for this boy's fatigue.

Another case illustrates the same principle with a not-so-obvious cause. Betty was a fifty-year-old bank clerk who complained of fatigue of about six months duration, and who could at first think of no obvious change in her life situation to account for it. More careful questioning revealed that she had joined the Y about the time of fatigue onset and had taken up jogging, which she had assumed would relieve some of her ennui. Although she seldom jogged more than a mile every other day, she was subconsciously attempting to get her time down to seven minutes, from a beginning nine and a half. Also she continued to rest no more than seven hours per night. She was told to add an hour of sleep and to be content with a nine-minute mile, whereupon her fatigue promptly disappeared.

3. The fatigue tends to disappear with forced vacations, such as minor illnesses or events that interrupt the work load.

4. The fatigue tends to be less noticeable on weekends, especially if a few more hours of sleep become available.

5. There is ordinarily no problem whatever in going to sleep, or with awakening during the night or too early in the morning. Such persons are commonly said to be able to "sleep through a storm."

6. There is usually no obvious maladjustment to the environment, at least of major proportions, that is the bank clerk loves her husband, the high school student likes school, etc.

7. The complainant commonly is unaware of how little time he is allotting to rest and recuperation, or how long and onerous is the work load carried.

8. There is commonly an assumption that eight hours sleep per night is the magic figure for everyone in all situations. Experimentation with an extra hour, or half hour, of sleep may yield surprising results. Commonly going to bed a half hour earlier and arising a half hour earlier makes a big difference, lending some credence to the old adage that an hour's sleep before midnight is worth two after.

Mental Fatigue

Contrary to physiologic fatigue, mental fatigue responds best to action, especially of a vigorous physical type. In fact rest may aggravate mental fatigue. Mental fatigue is very likely when the following features are present:

1. The task producing the fatigue is commonly of a monotonous or repetitive type requiring intense mental concentration, especially from a sitting position. Good examples are assembling electronic units, inspecting labels, sewing, driving, typing, operating a reject line, etc. Standing in one place (to perform a repetitive task), or moving about slowly in a confined area, do little to detract from such fatigue.
2. Headaches, neck pain, and eye discomfort are commonly associated with fatigue and tend to appear after a few hours of such labor. Such pains disappear with aspirin or exercise.
3. Mental fatigue tends to increase in almost direct proportion to the amount of time that has elapsed on the task at fault.
4. Several minutes of vigorous exercise, such as swimming, jogging, or cycling, work almost magically to offset the effects of such fatigue. Less vigorous diversions, such as a coffee break, a walk, or a stretch session, afford less complete and less lasting relief.

Emotional Fatigue

Emotional fatigue—fatigue of nervous origin due to nervous tension—commonly possesses features of both physical and mental fatigue. Depending on the balance between the various components at any one time, it may be best helped by rest, or it may be best helped by vigorous exercise. Thus, the tense, nervous person may be so shorn of sleep by insomnia that physical rest is greatly needed. Unfortunately, it is often difficult for the chronically tense individual to come by such rest without the aid of drugs, unless, as you shall see, he utilizes a program of vigorous exercise tailored to the individual. However, despite its intricate linkage with physical and mental fatigue, certain features tend to characterize fatigue of emotional origin:

1. Unlike fatigue of physical or mental origin, tension fatigue tends to improve as the day wears on and job duties tend to diminish.
2. The chronically tense individual is more likely to be as tired, or moreso, on awakening as he is at the end of the day. He may find the most difficult part of his day, in terms of fatigue, to be simply getting out of bed in the morning.
3. As a corollary to 2 above, the chronically tense person may feel most alive in the evening, after a habitual cocktail or two.
4. Careful questioning of a completely honest person commonly reveals a deep-seated job dislike or disinterest, either as a result of a square-peg-in-a-round-hole syndrome or of repeated frustrations or hostilities in connection with the job.
5. Friction may be commonly found to exist in home situations as well as work situations in such individuals. "One dog, many fleas."

6. Chronically tense individuals commonly return from vacations as tired as before they left, inasmuch as a goodly portion of their time is spent in anxious concern about what is happening "back at the ranch." Also, vacations are commonly packed, by such persons, with twenty-four hours of planned activity per day, this in an effort to garner all the "goodies" that time allows.

7. Such individuals may even harbor a guilt feeling during periods of relaxation, feeling that they should be utilizing every moment of their time to achieve some goal, either real or imaginary. Thus they are unable to utilize time off to its full R and R advantage.

8. Such persons commonly feel less fatigued on nonwork days—weekends when job pressures are allegedly not being applied.

9. Work loads are commonly carried over from office to home, from weekdays to nights and weekends. A professional carried a briefcase with him perpetually between office and home, home and office, although he worked only fitfully on its contents. The case was almost a fetish which signified an unbroken continuity between office and home.

10. Chronically tense individuals usually note that vigorous exercise has more to offer, in terms of relief of chronic fatigue, than any modality they may have chanced across. Most such persons, however, have never given adequate exercise a proper trial.

11. Chronically tense persons are notoriously poor sleepers. If they fall asleep readily, they commonly awaken two or three times during the night and have difficulty returning to sleep. Or they may have difficulty falling asleep. Or they may awaken quite early in the morning at four or five A.M. and be unable to go back to sleep.

12. Such individuals are commonly depressed, despondent, moody, and irritable. They are also perfectionistic and intolerant of errors in others, the sort of person often described as being impossible to work for.

13. Attention spans may be poor, and in older individuals, memory may fade. These persons are commonly poor listeners.

14. Poor general physical conditioning, with obesity, mild high blood pressure, poor exercise tolerance, and such is often quite evident.

PART TWO

The Management of Physiologic Fatigue

Again, you are reminded that this book is concerned with chronic, long-standing fatigue as opposed to acute fatigue. All of us are familiar with acute physiologic fatigue—the pleasurable tiredness that follows participation in an athletic event, the desire for rest that follows a day of manual labor, the pleasant weariness after a long cross-country tour on a bicycle, the warm relaxation that engulfs us when we stand before a roaring fire after a tour on the slopes. And you should be equally mindful of the renewal that comes with the two sine qua nons for relief of such fatigue—rest and refueling.

While chronic physiologic fatigue is more insidious and subtle in its onset, the same principles of causation and relief apply to it as apply to acute fatigue, except that mental and emotional components are much more likely to be important factors. In essence, chronic physiologic fatigue represents a state of imbalance between catabolic (destructive) and anabolic (constructive, restorative) forces of metabolism, in which demands on the organism have, over the long haul (days, months, years), come to outweight the forces of restoration. Hence the formula for correction of chronic physiologic fatigue seems simple enough: reduce physiologic demand and increase physiologic restoration. But first visit the doctor.

The Doctor Visit

Whatever the psychic or somatic complaint may be, the first step in elucidating its cause must be a visit to the physician. You should never assume that, simply because the odds are in your favour, fatigue is not of organic origin. Many times even a minor physical or organic problem, subject to easy remedy, is sufficient to cause a great deal of chronic fatigue, particularly if the life situation is highly stressful. For example, many women complaining of fatigue have a simple iron-deficiency anemia, easily demonstrated by a blood count, which responds quite readily to the administration of iron and proper diet. Many children with chronic fatigue may be suffering from a low-grade infection, or from a mild allergy, either of which is readily treatable. There may be mild hypertension, easily detectable and very responsive to simple measures such as weight loss and salt restriction and a proper exercise-rest routine.

The moral is that you should always, in an effort to solve your fatigue problem, begin with a careful medical examination. It is money well spent, and even if the exam reveals nothing, the proper first step has been taken, and you may then proceed with confidence to more positive measures.

Quite obviously the management of fatigue due to organic causes belongs strictly in the realm of the physician. In this regard, it should be pointed out that many so-called treatment failures of chronic fatigue are due to poor adherence of the patient to the physician's instructions, whether they be relative to the taking of a prescription, or to diet, rest, or whatever. Physicians are not miracle workers, and the success of treatment depends as much on the cooperation of the patient as it does on the skill and understanding of the physician.

Reduce Physiologic Demand

A prime example of the tired man under too great a physiologic demand is the individual who works all day in the hot sun at one job and then takes on another at night that lasts into the wee hours of the morning. One such person I knew worked the graveyard (midnight to eight A.M.) shift in an oil refinery and followed with a day shift running his own filling station. He made a nice living, but I never saw or heard him any way except tired. He had an unhappy family situation, incidentally, for which he was trying to compensate and from which he was trying to escape. To a degree he accomplished his purpose, but he paid the price of chronic fatigue.

There are obviously two routes open to reduction of the aggregate physical demands on an individual: (1) lighten the mean intensity of the demands, or (2) decrease the duration of the demands. In the case just mentioned, Bob could have helped his situation (reduced his physical demands) by either cutting down the time he spent at work (thus affording more hours for rest); or obtaining work that was less demanding physically. Obviously the former course is the more desirable, where possible, but family economics may dictate otherwise, in which event the latter course may be chosen. In instances of extremely long-lasting fatigue, in which the individual is approaching exhaustion, he may have to reduce his standard of living in order to be able to cut his working hours. This course, though difficult for many to accept, is far preferable to a general breakdown in health such as exhaustive fatigue can produce. Life, despite lower living standards, becomes much more enjoyable. This facet of load reduction is considered later in greater detail.

Further, it is mandatory that other sources of fatigue—mental and emotional—be attacked simultaneously with the physiologic sources. This, of course, applies to combatting any type of fatigue. For example, Bob, carrying as he did a physical work load of sixteen hours out of twenty-four, would have been much less fatigued if he had had a happy home life. Physical fatigue is ameliorated a great deal, in general, if coexistent emotional problems are solved. Thus in the management of any primary source of fatigue—physical, mental, or emotional—you must never neglect secondary sources.

Increase Physiologic Restoration (Rest and Refuel)

Rest and refueling are the two activities necessary to increase physiologic restoration. Let's take a brief look here before they are explored in detail in the following chapters.

Rest

What constitutes adequate rest to relieve fatigue revolves around the answers to a number of questions: What is the normal requirement for sleep? Is sleep absolutely necessary for physiologic rest? How long has fatigue been present? Is it acute or chronic? The first three chapters in this part discuss rest.

Refueling

The expenditure of energy requires refueling—the intake of proper nourishment. Good nutrition revolves around two basic aspects: the quantitative and the qualitative. Quantitative means caloric intake, and qualitative means the types and source of the calories. A few of the more pertinent areas in this field, as they apply to chronic fatigue, are touched upon.

Again, this book is not concerned with the nutritional aspect of acute fatigue, such as occurs after participation in a sports event. The necessity of replacing acute fluid loss and certain electrolyte (salt) losses under such circumstances is a subject of its own. However, many of the same principles apply, and it is with such principles that we are here concerned. The chapters in this part following those on rest discuss refueling.

CHAPTER 5

Sleep

A period of normal sleep in man occurs in a series of four to six sleep-dream cycles lasting about ninety minutes each. Each cycle lasts from the end of one dream period, as measured by rapid eye movements (REMs), to the end of the next. Such a cycle is one of the basic cycles of all mammals and varies in length with the metabolic rate of the species. REM sleep (during which there is complete loss of muscle tone except in the eye muscles) is preceded by non-REM (NREM) sleep that occurs in increasingly deeper stages, but during which muscle tone is retained.

Whatever interferes with this cyclic activity (drugs, tension, forced wakefulness, illness) interferes with the normal sleep pattern, and thus fosters fatigue.

Normal Sleep Requirements

Ask the average person on the street how many hours sleep are necessary to restore him (after a day's work) to a rested state, and he will most likely tell you eight hours. This notion probably stems from empirically determined mores and customs formed by the natural limitations of the twenty-four-hour day-night cycle. That is, in the days when cultures were basically agrarian in nature, man worked as long as daylight gave him opportunity—about twelve to fourteen hours of each twenty-four. Add to this two or three hours required to perform the other necessities of existence, such as eating, and one has remaining about eight hours in which to rest.

In actuality, there is nothing magic about eight hours rest, and many sleep scientists consider six hours total sleep quite adequate for the young and middle-aged adult. How rested a person feels after a period of rest depends as much on the quality of the rest as on the quantity (duration), that is, how deep was the sleep or was it uninterrupted?

Any number of famous surgeons whose days regularly began at 5:00 A.M. and ended after midnight continued productive lives well into their seventies. True enough, their work was not as physical as that of a railroad lineman, but it was considerably more so than the average desk worker. If chronic fatigue was their experience, it did not show in their work, and one would have to conclude from their achievements that it was not a major factor.

Moveover, sleep requirements of individuals vary with a number of physical factors—age, sex, climate, environment, to name a few. For example, during infancy and childhood, growth demands longer periods of rest (up to eighteen hours a day in the newborn). But in old age, the gradual deterioration of body and mind commonly leads to decreased sleep requirements (as little as five or six hours a day, commonly broken). In the in-between adult years sleep requirements are highly individualistic, so that what may be required by one individual to alleviate the fatigue of a day's work may be either too little or too much for another person of the same age and sex performing the same amount of work. How do you arrive at your individual requirements? Chiefly by past experience and by experimentation.

By the time you reach adulthood, you usually have a pretty good idea of the amount of rest needed to offset the fatigue of a normal day's activity. Also, if you can recall sleep requirements at twenty-five or thirty and are not an oldster (over sixty-five), you can use pretty much the same requirements as applied then. In the event you don't recall those figures accurately, it's simple enough to give trial runs to varying periods of sleep, taking care to ensure proper sleeping conditions—quiet, darkened room with good ventilation, and soothing music if it helps to lull you to sleep. By and large, it is preferable to start sleep periods after reasonable periods of wakefulness, for there may be an element of truth to the old aphorism "an hour of sleep before midnight is worth two after." For example, retiring at 11:00 P.M. and arising at 7:00 A.M. may produce better physiologic results than retiring at midnight and waking at 8:00 A.M., even though the same number of rest hours are involved. Also, shoot for regularity of the rest-action cycle. Don't force yourself to exhaustion with eighteen to twenty hours of work and then attempt to catch up on your rest at one fell swoop. It simply doesn't work that way. Whatever your most favorable cycle—sixteen hours of activity, eight of sleep; or up seventeen hours, down seven; whatever—find it and try to stay with it. Irregularity of the day-night cycle is one of fatigue's greatest allies. If, however, your sleep pattern is inadvertently interrupted, don't let temporary loss of sleep concern you. There is nothing debilitating about the loss of one or two nights sleep, and even total wakefulness for two or three days has no known harmful effects.

Alternatives to Sleep

In recent years it has been demonstrated in the laboratory that actual sleep is not necessary to relieve fatigue provided the rest period is characterized by total relaxation and total concentration on pleasant, stimulating, constructive thoughts. Such a state causes the expenditure of no more calories than when one is in a basal state, that is burning only those calories necessary to maintain basal body functions (temperature, respiration, food processing, and such), as during sleep. Such states are approached by certain techniques, such as yogi, but few people are expert enough in the art to subsist solely on that mechanism alone and abandon sleep altogether.

Chronic Rest Deficits

So much for acute fatigue—the fatigue resulting from a day's work. But what of chronic fatigue, the day-in, day-out, tired-all-the-time variety not relieved by what should be adequate rest periods maintained in a regular cycle? In such states, where physical fatigue is the primary factor, it is usually found that at some time in the past, the individual simply began cheating himself of the opportunity to rest adequately. That is, he began working longer hours than there were available rest periods to bring about restoration, and he did so repeatedly, over long, extended periods of time. Look at Figure 10. It is diagrammatic of the rest-action cycle characteristic of all higher forms of life.

THE REST-ACTION CYCLE

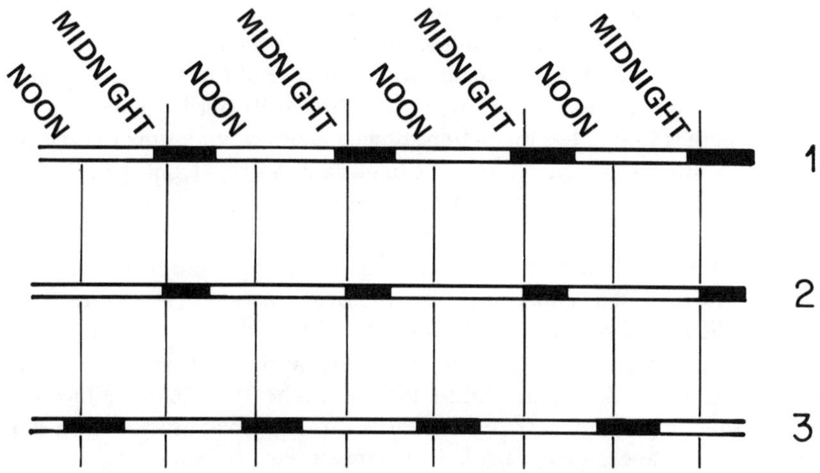

Black areas in bars are sleep periods. **White areas in bars are wake periods.**

Figure 10: The first crossbar illustrates a normal rest-action cycle, with a minimum of eight hours of sleep (required by most persons), at least two of which come before midnight. Note the regularity of the pattern.

The second bar illustrates a pattern in which the rest period is shortened to six hours. With most individuals such a pattern eventually leads to a chronic rest deficit and unavoidable fatigue.

The third bar illustrates the pattern of a night worker (midnight to eight A.M.) who sleeps in the daytime. Here the normal Circadian rhythm (the biologic clock) is inadvertently disturbed, with resultant fatigue.

Numerous other deviant patterns may occur, as with jet lag, irregular working hours, rotation of shifts, and so on. Any variation for long from the normal pattern usually leads to chronic fatigue.

If the proper rest-action cycle is ignored for sufficiently long (how long is highly variable from individual to individual, age to age, occupation to occupation, and so on) chronic fatigue results. One way to view it is that you can't take more money out of the bank than you put in and still stay in the black. And when the action phase of this rest-action cycle is habitually excessively prolonged by borrowing from the rest cycle, the result is, eventually, chronic fatigue. There is a point beyond which, unfortunately (and unlike the federal government), one cannot borrow without suffering dire consequences. Deficit financing simply won't work in the management of chronic fatigue. There comes a day when the bank must be repaid. The account must be balanced. And the only way to balance it is to rest.

It is my opinion that the habitual ignoring of this basic cycle as it applies to the human machine, over a period of years and years, so that the machine functions at a tired, low level of efficiency as a result of it, is responsible for the majority of the enforced rests that are brought on by superimposed disease states, such as coronary heart disease (heart attacks), stomach ulcers, colitis, high blood pressure, and a host of other diseases of civilization. The Sams of this world build their castles at the expense of their bodies, most of which, like a good horse, obey their rider (the will) until ridden into the ground. There is simply too much to be done and not enough time to do it in.

So the Sams go to their physiologic banks and borrow from their rest account until it is empty, and eventually they wind up in a hospital or a cemetery. The wise man, when made aware of this chronic imbalance, makes an honest effort to balance his account. Somehow, he goes to bed earlier and cuts his work load in any way possible. And over a period of weeks, months, and years, he is well repaid. But the fools, the Sams, do not take heed. They push on, their collective tongues hanging out, heedless of what their tired bodies are trying to say. They do, that is, until a heart attack or a bleeding ulcer or an artery "blowout" strikes them down in their tracks and sends them, via ambulance, to the bank to balance their account.

Getting to Sleep and Staying There

Knowing how much sleep you should have is one thing. Getting it is quite another. Assuming you are willing and able to shake up your old routine and get to bed earlier, how do you go about ensuring that extra time will be put to its intended use, sleep?

There's a solid rule of thumb that if a man can't go to sleep when it's time, he just hasn't "worked at it" hard enough, meaning that hard work (physically) is the best insurance available for going to sleep. And there's a lot of truth to that. Hard physical work or its leisure-time equivalent, exercise, are the best and most natural sleep-producers ever invented. There is more on this later.

But what if you have worked hard at getting sleepy, and when you hit the sack sleep doesn't come? Here are a few helpful hints on promoting that most natural of all bodily functions—sleep.

The Bedroom

Check the following items to see if your bedroom is conducive to going to sleep.

Light. Is the room sufficiently darkened, or is light creeping through from another room, or through the window? If it is, eliminate it. This may mean changing around an outdoor night-light, or putting up shutters—whatever it takes. Light is a stimulant to wakefulness. And darkness to sleep.

Temperature. Ideally the room temperature should be around 70° Fahrenheit. If the temperature is much above that and you can't bring it down, shed some clothes. If it's fixed much below that level, put some on or get some more cover. An electric blanket is an ideal means of maintaining proper body warmth in a cold clime. Proper body temperature is essential for going to sleep, and there is a rather narrow comfort zone in which sleep is more prone to come quickly. The next time you're fighting it, check on this one little item. Some fine adjustments can pay big dividends.

Noise. Quietude is basic to sound sleep. Although there may be a minority who have accustomed themselves to jungle rhythms from the squawk box as a prerequisite for going to sleep, the rule is that any level of extraneous sound, especially if it is nonrhythmical and atonic, is antisleep. Exceptions to this rule are the steady hum of an air-conditioner or a fan; here the noise is low-level, steady, and nonundulating, and may, in fact, be conducive to sleep in that it shuts out other types of sound. As a matter of fact, I have known some people who purposely run an electric fan in their bedroom for that very purpose, and they swear by it. Noises such as clanking machinery, dogs barking, or reverberating, drum-busting rock and roll are especially anathema to sleep. Briefly, the louder a sound the more likely it is to interfere with sleep. The louder, less musical, and more uneven a sound the more likely it is to sell sleeping pills.

Once in a while you'll find that person who can sleep in a boiler factory, or the kid who has to have the radio blaring when he sacks out, or the boob-tube enthusiast who can't turn it off unless the TV is turned on. Such cases are exceptions to the rule. They represent more of a conditioned response than a natural phenomenon. However, if absolute quietude isn't what you like to hear at bedtime, try soft, melodious music; or maybe even a boring TV show. But hook them to an automatic turn-off device so that a sudden change in program won't sound the alarm after you've gone to sleep. Some people have found metronomic devices, or even the tick of a grandfather's clock, to be sleep-producing. One would be foolish to insist that the shoe that fits one person's foot fits all. There's plenty of room for experimentation, and if you're one of those for whom sleep just won't come easy, despite adequate preparation, try your own thing.

It's a noisy world we live in, and when it comes to sleep, noise pollution has as much going against it as air pollution.

Air Circulation. Still air is stale air. And stale air is not conducive to sound sleep. For one thing, air must be kept in motion in order to keep it mixed so that a desirable temperature may be maintained. Again, stale air traps odors so that mustiness and disagreeable pungencies commonly result. In this regard, room airsprays, not used to excess, have a lot going for them.

While continuous air movement is desirable, strong drafts are to be avoided. They not only make accurate temperature regulation difficult, but may cause respiratory problems (soreness and dryness of the nose and throat, for example) which counter sleep.

As a rule modern air-conditioning systems afford the most ideal air circulation. Faulty installation may, however, pose any number of problems, of which proper circulation is only one.

Humidity. Ideal room humidity is ordinarily in the range of 30 to 35 percent. Most indoor room air is too dry, with humidity on the order of 10 to 15 percent (more dry than desert air), and too dry air causes drying of the mucous membranes, with resultant ill-effects. Excess moisture in the air is equally uncomfortable. Portable humidifiers are difficult to regulate. Centrally installed humidifiers, while expensive, are well worth the cost in terms of comfort conducive to sleep.

The Bed Itself. It's worthwhile to experiment with different sleeping surfaces. Those beds you get lost in commonly are conducive to aches and pains; firmer, orthopedic surfaces, generally speaking, give better body support. Ever try to sleep on a mattress that slopes toward the middle from all angles? You know what I mean.

If you're married and the initial honeymoon is over, you might try twin beds if your partner can't decide which side of the bed he is going to sleep on. And if the partner's snoring is a problem, more drastic measures may have to be taken. Having him stay awake until you get to sleep is not a very popular out, either. Such a problem may even call for a medical consultation, or separate bedrooms if the fatigue problem is severe enough to warrant it.

CHAPTER 6

Insomnia

Insomnia is a common bedfellow of chronic fatigue, so much so that it deserves special consideration. The chronic insomniac may either have difficulty falling asleep, or his nights may be punctuated with one to several episodes of wakefulness.

Insomnia affects millions of Americans, anywhere from 30 to 50 percent of the populace, depending upon its precise definition. The most common underlying causes are situational factors, medical conditions, psychological factors, drugs, and aging. Some of these have already been considered.

Management of Insomnia

In the management of insomnia, what not to do is as important as what to do. Let's look at some no-nos first.

Don't Use Stimulants

If you are taking a medication prescribed by your physician, you should apprise him of your insomnia. Some medications affect some individuals in a stimulatory manner (side effect), and it may be that your doctor can change the drug and cure your sleep problem. Any medication you are taking, whether by prescription or over the counter, should be scrutinized carefully as a potential cause of your pillow-pounding.

Much more commonly, stimulants are ingested in the form of food or drink, stimulants not ordinarily considered as such. The prime examples are coffee, tea, cola drinks, cocoa, and alcohol. If you are truly in earnest about ridding yourself of insomnia, these should be eliminated in their entirety.

Coffee contains caffeine, and caffeine is a potent central nervous system stimulant. More than one case of insomnia has been cured by the elimination of coffee from the diet. However, not all persons are similarly affected by coffee. Even if coffee drinking is confined to the A.M., in some persons it seems to exert a carry-over effect far into the P.M.If you are accustomed to taking four or five cups of coffee a day, cut down your intake slowly if you can't go it cold turkey. The first week cut your consumption by one cup per day, the second week by two cups, the third by three, and so on until you are on the wagon. Try substituting with decaffeinated coffee, vegetable or fruit juices, or just plain water. But don't expect the old urge won't be there for a while. It will. Not because coffee is addictive, but because you have become accustomed to the pick-me-up feeling coffee has given you. This is a feeling you can best do without, and with a little time and patience, the insomnia will be replaced by sound sleep, and in turn the early A.M. let-down by a relaxed, rested feeling. Chew gum. Chomp mints. Whatever. Just stick by your guns and before long you won't miss the brew at all. Some persons, unable to "hack" the cutoff, decide in favor of coffee and sleeplessness. Just remember that if insomnia is your problem, you may never lick it completely if coffee is your hangup.

Cola drinks, unbeknownst to many consumers, are another potent source of caffeine. A coke or two a day may well produce the same effect as coffee, especially if taken in the P.M. One physician drank cokes instead of coffee to wake up on and kept at it all day long. He slept very little, he said, but then he was one of those "human dynamos" who apparently didn't miss his sleep that much. Like coffee, these drinks should be verboten if you are determined to lick your sleep problem.

Tea contains theophylline, a compound very similar in structure and pharmacologic action to caffeine. Though not as potent a central nervous system stimulant, tea taken injudiciously nevertheless may have a very similar insomniac effect. Hence it, too, should join coffee as a no-no in persons who make a habit of counting sheep far into the night.

Likewise for cocoa, which contains theobromine, a chemical relative of caffeine which, though less potent a stimulant than either caffeine or theophylline, can produce insomnia especially if taken at bedtime, as it is commonly used (or misused) in an effort to promote sleep.

Say Goodman and Gilman in their text on pharmacology, "The earliest use of the xanthine beverages (coffee, tea, cocoa) is lost in the obscruity of the past. However, legends telling of their discovery reveal the reason for their favor. For example, legend credits the discovery of coffee to a prior of an Arabian convent. Shepherds reported to this prior that goats which had eaten the berries of the coffee plant did not rest but gamboled and frisked about all through the night. The prior, mindful of the long nights of prayer which he had to endure, instructed the shepherds to pick the berries so that he might make a beverage from them. The success of his experiment is obvious from the popularity of coffee today, a billion pounds being consumed annually in the United States alone (World War II years)."*

Tobacco, with its high nicotine content (0.5 to 8.0 percent), is also a culprit in insomnia, especially when indulged in during the evening and bedtime hours. Nicotine is a powerful stimulant of the central nervous system, although stimulation may be followed by depression when large enough doses are taken. Moreover, it has a complex action on the entire nervous system, so that the sum total effect may be difficult to predict in a given individual. The smoke of the average cigarette may yield several "treatment" doses of nicotine; that from a cigar may contain up to fifty times as much; fortunately only a fraction of this is absorbed.

*L. Goodman and A. Gilman, *The Pharmacological Basis of Therapeutics* (New York: MacMillan, 1975). By permission.

Although insomnia is a relatively minor side effect of smoking (when compared to its cancer-producing qualities and its role in heart attacks), still when sleeplessness is the immediate antagonist, the stimulant properties of the habit assume major proportions. There is no easy way to quit smoking, but the person in earnest about licking his sleep problem finds a way. And he probably incorporates, somewhere along the way, the judicious use of the right kind of exercise. Any number of good books and booklets have been written toward licking the nicotine habit. Two of them are listed here:

H. Brean, *How to Stop Smoking*
The Benjamin Co., Inc.
485 Madison Ave., New York, New York 10022

National Clearinghouse on Smoking
and Health Center for Disease Control
Help on Smoking Cessation
Atlanta, Georgia 30333

Unfortunately the proper place of vigorous exercise in combatting the tobacco and other drug habits has not yet come into full recognition. But there is ample anecdotal evidence that, given a choice between nicotine and the achievement of a high level of physical fitness, the determined individual, quite naturally (for nicotine and good endurance simply do not mix), tosses away the fags every time. He also, as you shall see, tosses away any other drug that impairs performance in his quest for a high level of well being.

Alcohol, contrary to popular opinion, is not a stimulant. Pharmacologically it is a depressant, although the euphoria and lack of inhibition it produces in smaller doses is commonly mistaken for stimulation. Alcohol's anesthetic properties give it a place between general anesthetics and hypnotic drugs. The importance of alcohol in the chronic fatigue picture is twofold: (1) its chronic use lessens the appreciation of fatigue, so that an already-tired individual may spuriously feel relaxed after imbibing, thus he temporarily fools his mind, but not his body; and (2) its depressant action has a hangover effect (so well known following excessive bouts of drinking) which carries over to the next day (if used in the evening), necessitating the use of stimulant drugs like coffee to counteract its effect. In other words, its depressant action indirectly brings about an increased use of stimulants, which in turn add to the insomnia problem. Certainly the problem drinker, perhaps the day-to-day consumer of a friendly drink or two, must, if he is to lick insomnia, face up to his problem. Again its solution is not easy, but at the expense of sounding repetitious, I have encountered too many one-time imbibers turned marathon runners—persons who gave up the bottle for the breathing, so to speak—to ignore the prime role that a truly good exercise program can play in licking this, as well as other drug habits.

Next comes a variety of prescription or over-the-counter drugs of the upper or downer type; drugs like dexedrine or its analogues on which to get up and get going; and drugs of the tranquilizer or sedative type with which to turn off the uppers. The person who has come to rely on such pharmacologic crutches has created a seesaw existence which finds him on top of a mountain or down in a valley. And fatigue, the result of overstimulation with stimulants or of overdepression with downers, is his constant companion. Again he must conquer this particular type of drug habit just as he must conquer tobacco, coffee, or alcohol excess. And again the role of a vigorous exercise program and of rearranged life patterns cannot be overemphasized. When it is recalled that the people of this nation spend millions of dollars on tranquilizers, sedatives, and stimulants, the search for healthy alternatives becomes all the more imperative.

We are, indeed, a drug-oriented culture which fashions our mornings and our days from stimulants and then resorts to depressants in the evenings to counter the stimulants and rock us to a disturbed sleep. We have manufactured the sun by which we arise, the moon by which we retire, and the hours by which we rest and play. But in so doing we have ignored that most fundamental of all timers—the physiologic clock—and the price for this is chronic fatigue. Drugs can never supplant the rhythm of nature—not without the exacting of a very dear price: tension, fatigue, inefficiency, even premature death. The average citizen of the so-called civilized nations of the world lives a life which, relative to the natural use of day and night, is as distorted as a pretzel. He has, over the years of his lifetime, so warped his work-rest cycle that he is hopelessly engulfed in physiologic debt from which he can never escape, never, I say, because he is unwilling and emotionally unable to pay the price of restoration to a semblance of normalcy.

How paltry few, indeed, how diseased, how inept, the fifty to sixty years our Sams warp into the molds of their own choosing and making, molds manufactured from a flaunting of every logical and reasonable law of diet, work, exercise, play, and rest. Civilization, indeed! Rather a complex, intricate, cunningly devised web of self-destruction.

The chronic fatigue which is so commonly experienced by the Sams of this world is, as we have seen, a manufactured item, just as certainly as autos are manufactured from steel. And drugs, of one or another type, are an integral part of its structure. If you are bent on conquering your fatigue problem, you must find a way to do without them.

Other Don'ts

It's an old saw that strong, visual stimuli, or more properly visual-emotional stimuli, are sleep antagonists. For some people, this is certainly true. For example, an episode of *Jaws* at bedtime would, for many, conjure up anything but sleep. The same can be said for exciting or horrifying radio programs, or even certain types of written material. On the other hand, the visual stimulation afforded by TV seems to exert a soporific effect on some people, even though blood is flowing and scalps are falling on the silver screen. And many can fall asleep faster on attempting to read *The Hound of the Baskervilles* than trying to wade through *War and Peace*. Music has much the same diversifying effect. What is a soothing, charming piece of music to one individual may so turn off another as to completely nullify its sleep-producing effect. In essence, the don'ts—don't watch, don't listen—which apply to any given individual at bedtime must be individualized. Find out what type of material turns you on, and then make it a point to avoid it at bedtime, just as you make it a point to know what turns you off.

Argumentative discussions are a no-no for evenings if sleep is your problem. Besides, many evening arguments are the result of daytime accumulation of fatigue, and a night's sleep pours oil on troubled waters. Likewise important decisions (as where considerable sums of money are involved, or where major changes in life are an issue) should be made *after* a good dose of sleep, and not when the mind is beclouded with fatigue. Decisions of some weight made in the evening often are second-guessed far into the night and provide just the irritant of thought that is likely to be a great hindrance to sleep. If you can train yourself to accept the fact that *sound sleep precedes sound decisions,* you have taken a giant step toward solving not only your sleep problem, but numerous others as well.

To any number of businesspeople, the briefcase carried home is a sign of success, and the briefcase left at the office signals sure failure. The home becomes a second office, where unfinished volumes of business pour over into evening hours. It is exceedingly difficult for many people to leave a typewriter or a brief or a thick shock of notes and turn at once to the business of sleep. As one wag put it, "the contents of my briefcase have a nasty habit of following me to bed." He said a mouthful, or an eye-openerful. If at all possible, you should leave your work at the office; if you *must* work after hours, you should do it at the office. The point is that your home should come to signify a place where work ends and rest begins. Over a period of time, home becomes a psychologic refuge as well as a physical one.

A most successful physician, a real genius with money, practiced this cardinal principle: business was never carried on, even discussed, within the confines of his home. If he had business to be done, it was done wherever necessary, but not at home. The moment he stepped into his house, it was relaxing music and reading. I never knew a more successful doctor, one who carried on at least three times the business activity of the average physician. During the daytime he was a veritable dynamo of activity; but when the front door to his home closed behind him, relax was the name of the game.

For a lot of people, better organization of one's day would solve the problem. But for those who find it impossible to leave the office at the office, it should never be business as usual right up to bedtime, topped off with a sudden effort to go from reams to dreams. Time must be allowed for a buffer zone between quitting time and retirement time, time in which relaxation is the theme and preretirement activity (see below) is the menu. Going through such a process is much more likely to meet with quick sleep than a quick flip from the pencil to the pillow. In summary, where at all possible, *do your work at the office; don't take it home.* If you must take your work home, *knock if off in time to prepare for sleep.* And, finally, *never, never take your work to bed with you.*

A.M. versus P.M.

Some persons find it difficult to awaken early, and their mental processes don't get into high gear until the P.M. Such P.M. persons would do better to arrange their work load so that it falls during the P.M., even arranging for later arising than most people and making allowances for later evening hours. For A.M. persons, the reverse is true. It's "early to bed and early to rise" that gets the job done for them. It just may be that a part of your fatigue problem relates to this physiologic variation from person to person. A bit of experimentation with different work-rest cycles might prove to be a real eye-opener, or should we say eye-shutter?

Some Do's for Sleep

Preretirement. The bedtime snack has long been a standard bit of activity calculated to promote sleep. Chances are that it's worthwhile *if* it's just a snack—a glass of milk, a bit of fruit, a cookie or two. But not if it's a Dagwood's Delight. Most of us would do better to put padlocks on the refrigerator and give away the key. Overeating is a part of the great American way, and overeating at bedtime is an invitation to sleeplessness or, at best, restless sleep.

The shower or bath is another time-honored point of departure for slumberland. Should it be hot or cold? As with other items, it's an individual thing. The warm shower followed by a good towel-down is most commonly accepted, but the cold shower followed by a quick transfer to a warm bed works wonders for others. More recently massage-type showerheads have added a new wrinkle, or should we say sprinkle, to the shower business. What it all boils down to is that you should try different techniques and combinations: shower versus bath, heat versus cold. Find out which is *your* "bag."

Mild exercise preceding the shower is worthwhile in some cases. You should not go in for sweat-production, but calisthenics of the muscle-stretching variety—a few knee-bends, sit-ups, and ceiling-touches (reaching high)—are sufficient. Contrary to popular opinion, such exercises promote muscle relaxation rather than tension and, if engaged in lightly, are quite conducive to quick dreaming.

Massage has already been mentioned. A sympathetic spouse with a good vibrator can work wonders with tensed-up muscles, and there's no better time for this than on retiring. Massage-beds (vibrators) or chairs have some strong proponents, but are fairly expensive and hardly necessary except in extreme instances.

Retirement. When you hit the sack, try some rather monotonous reading material for a turn-off. And turn on some good, soft music. In this regard, an automatic switch for turn-off is terrific. And your bed-light should be easily accessible. If you have to stretch a country mile to turn it off, you can undo a lot of preparation for sleep. It's the little things that can make the difference between quick success and prolonged parrying for sleep. If everything has been done correctly, you should fall asleep quite readily within ten or fifteen minutes (at the most) after you douse the light. If you have to turn more than two or three times you may be in for some tossing, and the following group of exercises (designed to consciously relax muscle groups in succession) may come in handy:

1. Lie flat on your back without a pillow, legs slightly apart, arms comfortably outstretched. Take several deep breaths, exhaling and inhaling deeply.

2. Scalp muscles: You may be surprised to notice, when you become consciously aware of it, that you are frowning. Counter this by deliberately raising the brows and holding them raised until it begins to feel uncomfortable. Then slowly relax them. You should be able to feel the scalp "loosen."

3. Facial muscles: Again it may surprise you that your mouth is "tied down" at the corners, or your lips tightly pursed, your jaws set. Force a big smile or grin, ear to ear, holding it to the point of mild discomfort. Then slowly relax. Let the jaws fall apart.

4. Neck muscles: Lift your head and hold it off the bed until discernible fatigue sets in. Then abruptly relax so that your head falls back to the bed. "Flop it" from side to side a few times.

5. Arms: Deliberately "stiffen out" the arms, fists clenched tightly, and hold them tensed for a minute or so. Then let them naturally relax and the fists unclench. Do this several times.

6. Legs: Deliberately stiffen and straighten out the legs as tightly as you can for a half minute or so. Then abruptly relax. Repeat several times.

7. Abdomen: While stiffening out the legs as in 6, lift them a few inches from the bed and hold this position as long as you can. Then abruptly let them drop as you relax the leg muscles. Repeat several times.

At first, you may have to go through the procedure two or three times. The idea is not only to induce total relaxation, but to get the feel of relaxation.

Unwanted Interruptions. Plenty of insomniacs have no problem turning it off rather promptly at sack time. But after an hour or more of sound sleep, their eyes pop open like corks erupting from a champagne bottle. What to do when this happens?

Well, you can try the old relaxing routine again. Or the soft music bit. Or at thirty minutes and counting, perhaps a small glass of juice or warm milk. If nothing seems to work, don't fight it. Turn on the light and pick up a book. Or if your train of thought runs to business matters inadvertently, pick up that notebook and pencil you should keep handy and do some fast and fancy jotting. That way you won't spend another thirty minutes trying to remember what got you awake in the first place.

Commonly when one yields to the insomnia—acknowledges it and "rolls with the punch"—sleep returns promptly. It's that old "I'll lick it or bust" attitude that starts the adrenalin to flowing. Many a goodly bit of knowledge has been gleaned from books in the middle of the night; in fact correspondence courses, study courses, whatever, have been passed with flying colors by the insomniac who uses the occasion of wakefulness to make hay, so to speak. As a matter of fact a goodly portion of this very book has been compiled or written in the wee hours when sleep was as elusive as a greased pig. Mind you, this is not a refutation of the "no business at night" theme a few pages back. Such madness should be a last resort, and you should have exhausted all reasonable means of returning to sleep before throwing in the towel (or should we say pillow?).

Oddly enough, you'll likely find that the next day you feel no more tired (if as much) when you learn to utilize those waking hours as when you lie there and fight it by the hour. Try it. You might like it. At least you'll have a feeling of accomplishment to buoy up your tiredness the next day. And the following night you'll most likely not wake at all.

Exercise. As stated previously, if sleep is hard to come by—so hard that you find yourself resorting to all sorts of tactics—chances are you aren't working your body hard enough. That is to say you can stand to increase your exercise output. Any number of marathon runners were insomniacs before they became runners. There is good evidence that physical exercise is a far superior mode of relaxation after a stressful day than a "drunk" or sedatives. For example, the effect of alcohol in relieving tension is only psychological (forming a veneer over the underlying tension), while the effect of exercise is physiological. There is more to say about this later.

CHAPTER 7

Recreation and Vacations

If a life pattern consists only of the rest-action cycle, or rather the rest-work cycle, Jack becomes more than just a dull boy; he becomes a dead boy at a ripe young age. Sleep alone does not fill the bill for recharging the batteries of life. Recreation and vacations are necessary.

Recreation means "to create anew," to do a new thing. Recreational activity occupies that portion of leisure-time not spent in performing the necessary things of life (eating, sleeping). Such activity is as important a phase of rest as is sleep itself. The galley slave, chained to his oar, existed in a work-sleep pattern devoid of recreation, and died at an early age. Similarly, the slave to his work, any type of work, who has no time for play or diversion, is an almost certain candidate for chronic fatigue and perhaps premature death.

Recreational activity may take many forms—from midday siesta to listening to Bach to bird-watching to jogging to sipping a soda—whatever affords a turning away from the rut and routine of life. It may occupy a few minutes (coffee break) to an hour (noonday break) to a few days (weekends) to weeks or months (vacation). Whatever its form or however long a period of time it occupies, in the combatting of chronic fatigue it deserves special attention.

In one sense—the sense that play is often involved—recreation is a reversion to childhood, with freedom from the responsibility of making a living or carving a niche. It is as essential to the total well-being of man as food or drink. The more absorbing and engrossing it is, the more it shields us from the stress of life, and the more it renovates, or restores, the haggard mind and body.

Such forms of recreation as coffee breaks were long ago recognized to increase the efficiency of workers, especially those engaged in sedentary activity. More recently, exercise breaks have been shown to produce even better results in workers doing monotonous and repetitive tasks not of a strenuous nature. In general, persons engaged in vigorous livelihoods (requiring intense muscular endeavor) seek more sedentary types of recreation and vice versa. For example, the construction worker might understandably prefer fishing to jogging, while the desk worker might easily prefer tennis, though there is no reason that a variety of recreational activities cannot be indulged in by the same individual. Variety is indeed the spice of recreation.

Whatever else may be said of him, the successful fatigue-fighter utilizes one or several recreational outlets. He does not only dare, but finds it essential, to become a child again for a little while each day. He is his own expert at something that does not fit into the workaday world: tennis, painting, coin-collecting, bird-watching, fishing, or just watching and comparing sunsets. For in the wise use of recreation true values are to be found, more so even than in the hard ruts of life. It is beyond the dollar sign and the mortgage payment and the time schedule and the telephone, those inexorable factories of fatigue, that the essence of being alive is found. Fatigue is released when a man learns to assess his true size beside an ocean and to see a universe in a grain of sand; to realize that, indeed, life's greatest treasures are to be found outside the bank vault.

Gold dust on a monarch's wing,
    Spun silver on a lake's quiet breast,
Dew-diamonds all aglow at morning,
    These—these are my treasure chest.

When I had been in medical practice for but a few months, I was riding down a hospital elevator with an older practitioner who had been in practice for many years. It was summertime and the subject of vacations arose. "I'm headed for two weeks in Florida," he said joyfully, "and you?"

"Can't afford time off," I said. "Too much red ink."

"Young man," he said, "listen good. You can't afford *not* to take a vacation. And don't forget it."

Well I haven't forgotten it, and there have been times when I really couldn't afford time off because of red ink, or last-minute complications. But I have always gone ahead and taken it. And in the long run it has proved an investment that has paid off well. My only regret is that I haven't wangled more vacation time than I have!

Vacations, wisely planned, afford a time not only for rest and recreation, but for backing off and taking a long look at the overall pie, where you've been, where you're headed, and what for. This means time for meditation in a rested state. Unfortunately the great majority of vacationers see the vacation period as a brief interlude into which as many as possible things to do, things to see, and places to go should be packed into each and every day and night. There is no time for utter and complete relaxation; that's a waste of precious time. The end result is a vacationer who is as tired when he returns from his trip as when he left, if not more so; a vacationer who must plunge back into the same maelstrom that he left without so much as a chance at a new perspective. In effect, he has stepped off his merry-go-round just long enough to run pall-mall around the block and climb back on again.

All this is not to knock sight-seeing and doing things for which there is no opportunity at other times, but it is to knock the militaristic schedule that crams a two-week program into a week, or a month into half a month. If the vacation you are looking at plans every hour of your day for you, forget it as far as relieving fatigue. You're far, far better off renting a canoe and floating down the nearest river. See that your plans leave ample time for doing simply nothing, just as you please, or tear them up and start over.

The doctor I mentioned in the first paragraph of this subject was a veritable fireball at work, he could do more in a day than most doctors could in two. But he knew how to relax. He could fall asleep between a woman's labor pains while awaiting a delivery, and when he went to Florida he didn't try to take in all the scenery in a mad race with time. He found a nice corner of the beach and staked out a claim and listened to the waves and the wind. He took a big dose of what he didn't have time for back in the rat race, and he told me he always felt like a new man when he did. And when he began to feel run down at the seams, he made time for another dose of the same kind of medicine—a big dose of nothing. The moral is. if you're tired, dog tired, and there's no obvious reason, take as many days off as you can manage and plan to do a whole lot of nothing. Enough somethings-to-do always crop up to break the monotony, if any, and you'll have a welcome opportunity to take that long and needed look at tomorrow.

CHAPTER 8

Nutrition: Quantitative Aspects

Ideal Weight

The person at ideal weight should take in only enough calories to replace the daily loss caused by basal metabolic processes and the day's activities. What is an ideal weight? It is that weight which represents the proper ratio of fatty tissue to nonfatty tissue (muscle, bone, and internal organs). In other words, it is that weight which, for a given height and body build, you weigh when you are not obese and not undernourished. How do you determine if you are obese? There are several methods, none 100 percent accurate.

The simplest and most often-used method is to refer to height-weight tables such as those in the appendix of this book. Here a consideration of body build is important—whether one is lean and tall (ectomorphic), muscular (mesomorphic), or round-featured and paunchy (endomorphic). Body types are hereditarily predetermined, and one cannot and should not attempt to convert one type into another. Another method for determining obesity is by measurement of skin folds, using skin calipers and referring to a set of norms. This is usually best done by a physician or physician's assistant. Other methods involve the determination of a "ponderal index"* or suspension of a person by special weighing apparatus in a large tank of water (body density). Many such methods are used only experimentally, being too costly and too ponderous for routine use. Height-weight tables and skin-fold measurements are the two most commonly used methods, and afford a good point of departure in determination of your weight status.

Assuming your weight is ideal, how do you determine what your daily caloric intake should be? Obviously, if you have gotten along for years and maintained the same ideal weight without reference to tables and measurements, you don't need to give too much special attention to this facet of your diet. You're doing okay more or less by instinct. There are several methods, however, to determine your daily caloric intake:

1. Some simple arithmetic: Multiply your weight in pounds by fifteen (if an adult). The product gives you roughly the number of calories per twenty-four-hour period needed to maintain that weight.

*The ponderal index may be determined by dividing your height in inches by the cube root of your weight in pounds. Ponderal indexes below 12.3, and especially 11.6, are commonly (but not always) associated with significant obesity. Example: John weighs 150 pounds; his height is 6 feet (72 inches). His ponderal index is therefore 72" divided by 5.3 The cube root of 150), or 13.6, an index of non-obesity.

2. Count calories: There are any number of sources—diet books, books on nutrition, calorie counters—that list the caloric content of a given helping of food. By jotting down the food items you ingest each day, meal by meal, item by item, and setting down opposite them their caloric content, you can total your caloric intake at day's end. Do this for seven days and take an average. This gives you your average daily caloric intake.

3. Consult tables: For example, a rough idea of your daily caloric requirements may be obtained from the following (for adults):*

Sedentary work—	1800-1900 calories
Light activity (business and professional)—	1900-2400 calories
Moderate activity (mechanics)—	2400-2800 calories
Heavy activity (laborers)—	2800-4500 calories

The Obese Individual

Obesity means excess weight due to fat. Ordinarily body fat constitutes no more than 15% of body weight, if an adult is not obese and a male, or 18- to 20 percent if a female. When body fat content exceeds this, obesity becomes a problem in many ways. *Where fatigue is the problem at hand, obesity must go!* Why? Consider the following:

1. *Extra fat is a "pack on the back."* Due in large measure to the fact that extra weight requires extra calories, the obese individual usually eats what amounts to four complete meals a day instead of three. Very simply, a larger energy supply is required to carry the extra load; and if a fat person's activity consists of more than sedentary duties, the extra caloric requirements are magnified many times. In order to meet these extra requirements, the obese person's heart rate increases, as does his respiratory rate, even at rest. When such a person is required to work, breathlessness commonly results. An obese person's respiratory rate exceeds the nonobese individual's by about three times per minute, an extra 4,400 respirations per day. His resting pulse rate commonly exceeds that of the nonobese by ten beats per minute, or about fourteen thousands beats per day. With increased pulse rate the work of the heart is, of course, increased concomitantly.

These requirements are present in an indolent person; they may be multiplied many times when a fat person becomes active. The effect is the same as if a normal-weight person straps an extra pound on his back for each pound of fat, and carries it with him wherever he goes, day in and day out. Make you tired to think about it? If it doesn't, try thinking of fifteen pounds extra, fifty, one hundred. The 150-pound person who is 10 percent overweight (minimal), for example, packs an extra fifteen pounds. If he is 30 percent over, he packs forty-five pounds. The first thing a tired mountain climber does when he stops to rest is take the pack off his back. If fatigue is your problem, losing the fat pack may be number one on your list.

*These figures are for persons of average height and weight.

SAMPLE PAGE FOR DAILY CALORIC INTAKE RECORD*

Date: Food or Drink Item	Portions (teaspoons, slices, cups, etc.)	Calories per Portion		Total Calories per Item*	Total Calories per Meal
		Breakfast			
Bacon, fried	2	50	=	100	
Egg, poached	1	100	=	100	
Bread	1	64	=	64	
Milk, skim	1	87	=	87	
Orange juice, fresh	1	108	=	108	
					459
		Lunch			
Tuna sandwich	1	350	=	350	
Potato chips	12	11	=	132	
Tea	1	0	=	0	
Sugar	1	16	=	16	
Sherbert	½	118	=	118	
					616
		Dinner			
Lettuce	½ head	30	=	30	
Mayonnaise	1 T	100	=	100	
Flounder	4 oz.	78	=	78	
Asparagus	6 spears	22	=	22	
Milk, skim	1	87	=	87	
Carrots (1/3 cup)	1	15	=	15	
Bread, whole wheat	1	55	=	55	
Margarine	1 T	100	=	100	
Cookies, plain	2	100	=	100	
					687
		Total Calories per Day			1762

**See calorie counter.

2. *Obesity breeds undesirable bed fellows.* The incidence of high blood pressure and diabetes is considerably higher in obese populations. Sustained high blood pressure develops at least two or three times as rapidly as in the nonobese. The same is true for diabetes and for atherosclerosis. Aside from the premature aging and death commonly associated with these problems, they commonly beget fatigue, which is our present concern. A goodly percentage of diabetics and mildly hypertensive persons, when overweight, revert to normalcy by the simple expedient of losing excess fat.

Obese persons don't like mirrors. As a group obese individuals don't like what they see in the mirror. They have poor self-images, and often quite distorted ones. And poor self-images lead to poor interpersonal relationships, which in turn lead to dejection, despondency, depression, and fatigue. Your psychological estimation of yourself is important in determining your overall sense of well-being. And tying a bulge of fat on your midriff is the psychologic equivalent of smearing pie on your face. You'd rather not flaunt it in public. As you lose fat, you feel better. You move better. You become, in a very real sense of the word, a different person.

4. *Obesity begets laziness.* The phrase "fat and lazy" contains more truth than poetry. And laziness heaps more fuel on the fires of futility and frustration. The lazy person, if not already so, commonly becomes an underachiever. Underachievement, a feeling of inability to cope successfully with one's environment, leads to feelings of fatigue. Thus a vicious cycle is established, and the longer it "wheels" the more difficult it becomes to break.

Incidence of Obesity

When you realize that obesity affects at least 25 to 30 percent of the adult population of this country (depending on where you draw the line between obesity and normalcy), you rightly arrive at the conclusion that a fair portion of the total fatigue problem is in some measure linked with obesity. Indeed many of the problems and life situations which lead to obesity also lead to fatigue—emotional conflict, frustration, depression, and so on. Combatting emotionally induced fatigue is dealt with in the next part, but as is obvious, whether it be the *cause* of fatigue or an *end result* of complex life situations which produce fatigue, obesity is equally undesirable and must be dealt with accordingly.

Although at least 95 percent of obesity cases are exogenous in origin—resulting from habitually ingesting more calories (stored as fat) than are used up—any serious reducing program should begin with a visit to the doctor to rule out one of the 5 percent causes which might require medical treatment.

How Fat Is Fat?

How do you determine your degree of fatness? As has already been shown, you may refer to height-weight tables or to skin-fold measurements or to the more erudite methods where these are available. If, for example, a male of medium build, 5 feet 10 inches tall, weighs 180 pounds, he (by reference to tables) is twenty pounds overweight. Thus he is 12.5 percent (twenty pounds divided by 160 pounds) overweight. His weight (180 pounds) is 112.5 percent of ideal (112.5 x 160 = 180).

From the standpoint of disease or longevity, the cut-off point for doing something about obesity is at the 25 to 30 percent level. In other words, fighting fatigue demands a sterner dealing with obesity than does the problem of organic disease. Thus if a chronically tired person is 15 percent or more overweight, he should attack his avoirdupois. The tolerance factor for overweight when fatigue is the problem may actually be less than that when organic disease is the prime consideration.

Fighting Fat

How do you get rid of fat? It isn't easy, and it is not a one-time deal. As a matter of fact, a number of things have been learned about obesity in recent years, the most important of which follows:

1. Obesity is a lifelong problem which, like diabetes, can only be controlled, not cured. You do not lose a few pounds, or even many, and then resume your precontrol habits without paying the price of recurrent obesity. There is good evidence that heredity plays a strong role—obese parents are more likely to have obese children.

2. Lifetime control implies lifetime effort. One must thus learn, accept, and maintain a new way of life and abide by a new set of rules—*from now on!*

3. Education in the ways and means of calorie counting, both as to input and output, is basic. The educational process is not a one-time thing, but an ongoing one that requires, in the early stages, close contact between you and professional advisors (physician, dietitian, nutritionist, physical educators).

4. The most satisfactory diet is a sensible, well-balanced one which represents a change in quantity, not quality. There are no super diets or magic formulas. Crash diets, starvation, and the like, if used at all (in exceptional cases) should be undertaken only under strict medical supervision. As a rule, slow, steady weight reduction yields better results than the more dramatic crash programs.

5. Drugs, such as hormones or diet suppressants, are, in primary obesity (not secondary to some other disease), only crutches that are best left unused. In children especially they are a no-no.

6. If there is a strong emotional component to the problem, it must be ferreted out and corrected.

7. The treatment of obesity requires intensive, prolonged contact between you and those involved in your care.

8. The use of physical exercise in conjunction with diet is a far more physiologic, sensible, and satisfactory approach than is diet alone.

9. Physical activity must be increased gradually but steadily at every possible opportunity. Sedentary activity is for the obese an outright luxury.

10. A program of physical activity tailored to the patient is as important an aspect of management as the restriction of calories.

From facts such as these, it becomes evident that fighting fat is a lifetime battle. Reduced to its simplest formula, fat-fighting involves a reversal of the formula for gaining weight, which is:

Caloric intake is greater than caloric output = Calories stored as fat. Reversal obviously requires:

Caloric intake is less than caloric output = Calories lost as fat.

There are three ways in which this weight-loss formula can be activated:

1. Decrease caloric intake while caloric output remains the same.
2. Increase caloric output while caloric intake remains the same.
3. Increase caloric output and decrease caloric intake simultaneously.

The third of these is the most physiologic route to go and, at least theoretically, may double the rate of weight loss as follows:

Example: Steve weighs 180 pounds and should weigh only 150. He is therefore thirty pounds or 20 percent overweight. Since each pound of fat represents 3,500 stored calories, he therefore has 105,000 calories (30 x 3500) stored as fat.

If he chooses plan 1 above (decrease caloric intake; output same), and goes on a diet which cuts his caloric intake per day by 1000 calories, he requires roughly 105 days (three and a half months) to reach ideal weight.

If he chooses plan 2, choosing to expend 1,000 more calories per day while retaining the same caloric intake, the time required would be the same. (Such an output, incidentally, represents jogging for about one and a half hours, covering perhaps ten miles daily, a terrific output attained by very few people).

By choosing plan 3—combining 1 and 2—he accomplishes the same result with considerably less misery. Say, for example, he reduces his caloric intake by 500 calories (not nearly so difficult to do as cutting it by 1,000) while at the same time he expends an extra 500 calories per day (still a goodly blow, but again, not nearly so difficult as with plan 2).

Over the long haul, in particular, a combination of sensible dieting and exercise pays off far more handsomely than attempting to utilize either diet or exercise alone, and it is much more physiologic. Foremost authorities on obesity control favor this technique. The individual who learns to control his weight by utilizing both diet and exercise has a far better chance to stick with it and establish a lifelong pattern than the dieting nonexerciser. Relapse rates from dieting alone are high—85 percent or so. It's an on again, off again sort of thing most of the time. When sensible exercise is introduced into the program, relapse rates are reduced considerably, because it's an easier and more acceptable row to hoe.

Here, in outline form, is presented a method of obesity control which I have used in practice for a number of years:

Step 1: Determine ideal weight.

Step 2: Determine pounds and percent overweight (actual weight-ideal weight and pounds overweight ÷ ideal weight)

Step 3: Determine rate of weight loss (subject to variation)
If: 10-19 percent overweight, 1/2 lb per week
20-29 percent overweight, 1 lb per week
30-39 percent overweight, 2 lbs per week
40-49 percent overweight, 3 lbs per week
50 percent or more overweight, strict medical supervision.

Step 4: Determine average daily caloric intake (DCI) at present weight. If adult, multiply weight by 15, or: consult calorie counter and keep item-by-item record, day by day, of calories consumed for one week. Add the seven days' intake and divide by 7 to get average. Use this counting method for children also.

Step 5: Lop the necessary number of calories off your DCI to effect the desired rate of weight loss (Step 3).
Remember: 1 lb. of fat stores 3500 calories.
So: To lose 1 lb. of fat per week, one must consume 3500 less calories per week, or 500 less per day (3500 ÷ 7)
To lose ½ lb. per week, ½ that much (250 less per day)
To lose 2 lbs. per week, 2x that much 1000 less), etc.

Step 6: Take up a leisure-time activity (LTA) that:
1. Starts slowly.
2. Increases gradually in intensity or duration.
3. Utilizes the large leg muscles.

Examples are walking, swimming, jogging, bicycling, mountain climbing, sculling (and game variations such as tennis, soccer, and basketball if not relied on entirely).

Outline a program (by consulting charts that list caloric costs of these activities)* in which you start out by using up 100 calories a day in this activity and gradually, but steadily, increase your caloric output to the 500-or-more-per-day level, or at least as far as your physical condition permits (see below).

If you are already engaging in one of these activities and still have a weight problem, you need to step up your caloric output and step down your caloric intake.

As your LTA increases in duration and intensity, you may let up on your caloric restrictions, so that if, for example, you are lopping 500 calories per day off your intake, you may lop off only half that (250) if you increase your LTA by 250 calories.

You should never, under any circumstances, start a vigorous exercise program to which you are unaccustomed without first consulting a physician and stating clearly your intentions. Not all persons entering a fitness program can or should attempt, by any

* See Appendix 2

> means, to become a marathon runner. On the other hand, there is a right amount of exercise, both as relates to intensity and duration, for practically everyone, regardless of age, in most cases.
>
> In controlling weight the *total calories used up* in a given activity is the important thing. Whether this is accomplished in twenty minutes of jogging or one hour of walking is irrelevant. Calorically the end-result is the same.

Over a period of weeks, months, or even years in some rare instances (if one doesn't get bowled over by that old bugaboo discouragement), weight normalizes or reaches the acceptable range, at which time the faithful fat-fighter should have achieved a feeling for his routine. This is to say that he can sense excessive caloric intake and almost instinctively cut it down or step up caloric output (LTA). Records and charts, once this level has been achieved, are unnecessary. LTA should, by this time, have become so habitual a thing that to miss it is like forgetting to brush one's teeth at day's end.

What has been established, at this level, is a new way of life that instinctively and systematically and regularly limits caloric intake and utilizes caloric output so that ideal weight is a natural end product. Further it is a way of life that the owner would not trade for the old way. The multitudinous beneficial effects of regular exercise are so essential to long-term maintenance of such a program that you have to wonder how the fat-fighter who utilizes diet alone manages to stick it out as long as he does.

Obesity can be licked, but licking it requires a mixture of iron will, steely determination, and bulldog tenacity. Not only can obesity be licked, but for the chronically fatigued, it must be.

Psychologic Factors in Obesity

Much obesity results from psychological hangups and depression. Distorted body images are common. Following are a few "table rules for dieters" that take such facts into consideration. Much of the problem with the overweight person lies in his behavioral approach to foods. He tends to pounce on every ounce and devour his meals in record time, thus giving no time for his "satiety center" (in the brain) to turn off his hunger. Consuming 2,000 calories in ten minutes may leave such a person still hungry, whereas taking thirty minutes to consume half as much leaves that individual perfectly content. The following suggestions are designed to be of help in retraining your approach to food.

1. Don't come to the table angry, depressed, or out of sorts if you can possibly keep from it. Assume a cheerful attitude.
2. Put before you all the food that is to be consumed at that meal.
3. Plan five or six small meals, including a bed-time snack, instead of two or three large ones.
4. Place salads and desserts in separate dishes from the main item(s).
5. Allow at least thirty minutes for your meal. You may not use all of

it, but make it available, and t-r-y to s-t-r-e-t-c-h the meal over that length of time. Never eat on the run.

6. Sit down in pleasant surroundings when you eat. Never stand up while eating. A bouquet of flowers on the table or a seat near a window helps to divert attention from food.

7. Take small bites of food or only a swallow or two of your fluid at a time.

8. Chew each mouthful of food until there's nothing left to chew. Taste your food (exercise your taste-buds). Relish it. This can only be done by slow, almost lazy mastication.

9. Never preload your fork or spoon. Wait until your mouth is empty before reaching for the next bite. Put down your eating or drinking utensil between bites or swallows.

10. Practice leaving a bite or two of your favorite item behind. The "clean-plate kid" title should go to Skinny Joe, not to you.

11. If desired you may peruse light reading or picture material while you eat; or you may engage in conversation, preferably with someone in the same boat as you.

12. If you feel you just *must* have something else after you have finished eating (especially when first starting out), drink a tall glass of water *slowly*. You may find you've been missing something all along.

13. Between-meal snacking and nibbling and ice-box raiding are a definite no-no unless low-caloric tidbits, such as radishes or celery or carrot sticks, are used. An occasional low-calorie soft drink is permissible.

14. Do not leave food within easy reach or sight. Out of sight makes out of mind easier.

One further point deserves emphasis here. It has been pointed out that five or six small meals per day are better than two or three large ones, when it comes to fighting obesity. In this regard, the "snacker" has a great deal to be said for him. But even the normal weight person who has a fatigue problem should avoid large meals. Food must be digested, and this requires digestive work. The more food crammed into the stomach, the more work must be done to process it. And excessive work, even of a digestive type, produces fatigue. Thus the somnolence and apathy which follows a turkey dinner. Too many people in overdeveloped countries don't know what it is to leave the table when hunger has been satisfied, rather than when the gut has been sated. We suffer from malnutrition of the overabundant rather than the under type. In many, many ways, it's a dying shame.

About Diets

Nowadays practically every publisher has his own diet book. Some of the diets being utilized nowadays are harmful, even dangerous—crash diets which take off pounds at the expense of protein (muscle) rather than fat; and high fat/high cholesterol diets which, in susceptible persons, may add considerably to the risk of a heart attack. It is unfortunate that some such diets have enjoyed tremendous acceptance by the general public. Furthermore relapse rates by those employing such extremes of diet are very high (85 percent). It's on again, off again, rather than steady does it.

There are a number of very reputable and worthwhile organizations for taking off excess weight. Among these are Weight Watchers and TOPS (Take Off Pounds Sensibly). These organizations are well run and do a very creditable job, utilizing well-balanced diets and a slow, but more sure, technique than crash programs. However, exercise is not stressed, and again, relapse rates are relatively high.

As stated, the steady, combined use of diet and exercise in sensible proportions is the most physiologic and widely accepted (by medical authorities) method of reaching and maintaining ideal weight, and once ideal weight and a high level of fitness are attained, relapse rates are pleasantly low.

CHAPTER 9

Nutrition: Qualitative Aspects

The qualitative aspects of the dieter refer, in particular, to an optimum intake of (1) vitamins; (2) minerals; (3) the three major foodstuffs: protein, carbohydrate, and fat; (4) certain essential amino acids (protein building blocks); and (5) essential fatty acids.

Vitamins

Pure Magic

Two popular theses, neither of which is correct, seem to govern the use of vitamins nowadays: (1) vitamins are good for whatever ails you, and (2) if a little bit of a vitamin is good, a whole lot is better. Regarding the first of these, vitamins are dietary essentials that the body is unable to synthesize in its own metabolism and must therefore obtain from outside sources. And while they are essential to normal body functions they are most assuredly not a panacea for the ailments of man. It is more the rule than the exception that a patient with a chronic complaint of any kind—and certainly chronic fatigue—has tried vitamin therapy, self-prescribed, before he consults the physician. The vitamin craze is universal, and so long as they are taken in harmless amounts, they may even provide a psychologic crutch that is helpful to many persons.

In the second premise—a whole lot is better than a little—lies not only folly but potential danger. So-called megavitamin therapy—in which one or more vitamins are taken in huge quantities (many, many times the recommended daily allowance [RDA]) without demonstrable deficiency states—has currently come into fadism not only by the public but by some physicians as well. The danger is twofold: (1) the unsuspecting layman who prescribes huge vitamin doses for himself may produce irreversible disease states (hypervitaminosis), especially with vitamins A and D; and (2) physicians utilizing such therapy may unwittingly produce presently unrecognized disease processes which may not become evident until irreversible damage has been done.

The toxicity of *vitamins A and D* in large doses has long been known in medical circles. These vitamins can not only produce illness when taken like candy over prolonged periods, but can kill. In the case of vitamin D the toxic dose is on the order of only five to ten times the minimum amount necessary to prevent rickets; thus its margin of safety is relatively small. Short of causing severe disease, megadoses of vitamin D may result in bone and liver

VITAMINS*

How Much Is Recommended of Each Vitamin		Why Each Is Needed	Some Good Food Sources
Vitamin A		Helps to form and maintain healthy function of eyes, skin, hair, teeth, gums, various glands and mucous membranes. It is also involved in fat metabolism.	Milk, egg, hamburger, liver, peaches, carrots, margarine or butter
Infants	1500 I.U.		
1-4 years	2500		
Over 4	5000		
P and L**	8000		
Vitamin B_1 (Thiamine)		Helps get energy from food by promoting proper metabolism of sugars.	Milk, turkey, tuna, hot dogs, pizza, whole grain bread
Infants	0.5 mg.		
1-4 years	9.7		
Over 4	1.5		
P and L	1.7		
Vitamin B_2 (Riboflavin)		Functions in the body's use of carbohydrates, proteins, and fats, particularly to release energy to cells.	Milk shakes, eggs, cottage cheese, cheeseburger, whole grain bread
Infants	1.6 mg.		
1-4 years	0.8		
Over 4	1.7		
P and L	2.0		
Vitamin B_6 (Pyridoxine)		Has many important roles in protein metabolism. It also aids in the formation of red blood cells and proper function of the nervous system, including brain cells.	Ham, popcorn, beef, fortified cereal, string beans, bananas
Infants	0.4 mg.		
1-4 years	0.7		
Over 4	2.0		
P and L	2.5		
Vitamin B_{12} (Cobalamin)		Helps to build vital genetic material (nucleic acids) for cell nuclei, and to form red blood cells. Essential for normal function of all body cells, including brain and other nerve cells as well as tissues that make red cells.	Milk, hot dogs, beef, liver, instant breakfast, turkey
Infants	2.0 mcg.		
1-4 years	3.0		
Over 4	6.0		
P and L	8.0		

* Vitamin Information Bureau, Inc., 664 N. Michigan Avenue, Chicago, Illinois. Reprinted with permission.

**Pregnancy and Lactation.

Folic Acid Infants 0.1 mg. 1-4 years 0.2 Over 4 0.4 P and L** 0.8	Assists in the formation of certain body proteins and genetic material for the cell nucleus, and in the formation of red blood cells.	Soybeans, liver, lettuce, carrots
Pantothenic Acid Infants 3.0 mg. 1-4 years 5.0 Over 4 10.0 P and L 10.0	A key substance in body metabolism involved in changing carbohydrates, fats, and proteins into molecular forms needed by the body. Also required for formation of certain hormones and nerve-regulating substances.	Eggs, nuts, liver, kidneys
Vitamin D (including D_2 and D_3) 400 International Units for all ages	For strong teeth and bones. To help the body use calcium and phosphorus properly.	Milk, tuna, milk shake, salmon
Vitamin E (Tocopherol) Infants 5.0 I.U. 1-4 years 10.0 Over 4 30.0 P and L 30.0	To help form normal red blood cells, muscle, and other tissues. Protects fat in the body's tissues from abnormal breakdown.	Cheeseburger, mayonnaise, lettuce, fortified cereal
Vitamin K Need in human nutrition established, but levels not yet determined beyond the newborn period	For normal blood clotting.	Leafy-green vegetables
Niacin (Niacinamide) Infants 8.0 mg. 1-4 years 9.0 Over 4 20.0 P and L 20.0	Present in all body tissues and is involved in energy-producing reactions in cells.	Hamburgers, whole-grain bread, turkey, fortified cereal

**Pregnancy and Lactation.

VITAMINS (Continued)

How Much Is Recommended of Each Vitamin		Why Each Is Needed	Some Good Food Sources
Biotin		Involved in the formation of certain fatty acids and the production of energy from the metabolism of glucose. It is essential for the working of many chemical systems in the body.	Egg, string beans, peanuts, liver
Infants	0.15 mg.		
1-4 years	0.15		
Over 4	0.30		
P and L**	0.30		
Vitamin C (Ascorbic Acid)		To help form and keep bones, teeth, and blood vessels healthy. It is also important in the formation of collagen, a protein that helps support body structures such as skin, bone, and tendon.	French fries, bell pepper, lemon, strawberries, juices fortified with vitamin C, tomatoes
Infants	35 mg.		
1-4 years	40		
Over 4	60		
P and L	60		

**Pregnancy and Lactation.

problems, skin problems, hair loss, headache, blood abnormalities, and apathy and fatigue, this quite aside from lethal propensities when taken in high enough doses for a long enough time.

Vitamin C (ascorbic acid) is currently on the throne as king of prevention. In the wake of popularization by the noted Dr. Linus Pauling, mothers cram this vitamin down their children in an effort to prevent all sorts of ailments, imaginary or real. Adults eat it like popcorn. It is available as candied mints, sugar-coated pills, and in various and assorted colors and strengths. The best thing that can be said about this practice thus far is that it is difficult to reach toxic levels with vitamin C; however, evidence is beginning to surface that in megadosage (50 to 100 times the minimum daily requirement), it too may have deleterious effects.

Vitamin C, like B-complex, is not stored in the body, and this probably accounts in some measure for its greater margin of safety. In all fairness, there is enticing evidence that ingestion of this vitamin in doses several times greater than the RDA may have beneficial effects. It is when one gets into astronomical levels that potential dangers arise. There is no question that after periods of severe stress (burns, debilitating disease, even periods of great emotional trauma) the body utilizes vitamin C for repair in quite large quantities. Further research is necessary to delineate carefully the margin between beneficial and potentially toxic doses. Caution is the order of the day.

Like vitamin C, *vitamin B-complex* (B_1, B_2, B_6, B_{12}, niacin, pantothenic acid and pyridoxine, and folic acid) is not stored in the body, and like C, even large doses appear to be tolerated, with rare exceptions, without demonstrable ill effect. Niacin in megadoses can cause unpleasant flushing of the skin, but this effect is not in itself harmful. Vitamin B-complex is commonly ingested in huge quantities by athletes seeking to build muscle or put on weight, but beyond the point of meeting increased needs under these conditions, there is no evidence that really large doses are beneficial.

One gentleman became so fatigued he had to struggle to get out of bed in the A.M. Medical consultation yielded negative evidence of disease. Finally, in desperation, he visited a health-food store and came away with B-complex in the form of bran, yeast, and B-complex capsules, all of which he began ingesting on a regular basis. Within a week or two, he avowed, he was a new man. In cases of this type, it is difficult to prove the role of the vitamin. One must entertain the possibility of a deficiency, or of some defect in vitamin metabolism, but far more likely is the psychologic effect in such instances. Even so if the effect is a cure of the fatigue problem, perhaps the end justifies the means; at least the B vitamins apparently do no harm, other than to the pocketbook.

Vitamin E, like C, is a highly controversial vitamin. Whereas there is little evidence that this so-called fertility vitamin, in large doses, is responsible for the claims made for it in the treatment of high blood pressure and fatigue, there are some instances on record that it may have adverse effects on both these problems—aggravation of high blood pressure and the production of fatigue by the vitamin itself. Its use in large doses should be under the supervision of a physician, or at least the physician should be made aware that his patient is taking it on his own. The most erudite investigators of the day consider vitamin E "a vitamin looking for a good use."

What, then, constitutes an adequate vitamin intake under ordinary circumstances, that is in an individual who is not ill? The following chart gives pertinent facts for each vitamin, lists the RDA* made by the United States Food and Drug Administration in 1973, and gives a list of foods in which the particular vitamin is found in abundance.

Thus for ordinary purposes an adequate formula for a standard maintenance vitamin tablet or capsule (for adults) might include:**

Thiamine (B_1)	2 mg.
Riboflavin (B_2)	2 mg.
Niacinamide	20 mg.

*Recommended daily allowance.

**Based on H. Pollock and S.L. Halpem and The Committee on Therapeutic Nutrition of the Food & Nutrition Board, *Therapeutic Nutrition,* National Research Council.

Ascorbic acid (vitamin C)	60 mg.
Calcium pantothenate	10 mg.
Pyridoxine	2 mg.
Folic acid	0.4 mg.
Vitamin B_{12} (cobalamin)	6.0 mg.
Vitamin A	5000. I.U.
Vitamin D	500. I.U.

Inasmuch as some vitamins are ingested in the diet, the daily ingestion of a vitamin supplement containing the above constituents in the amounts indicated (or thereabouts) ensures that minimum daily requirements of all vitamins are met. (Vitamin K, having to do with blood coagulation, is manufactured in the intestine and need not be taken medicinally by healthy individuals. The need for Vitamin E has not yet been established.) Even in industrialized, well-fed societies such as ours, it is possible to come up short on vitamin intake if meal-planning is sloppy. For example, if you consume the following items in a day, you consume 2,240 calories, but you are deficient in ascorbic acid, nicotinic acid, and thiamine, among other things:

Breakfast: 3 hot cakes with butter and syrup
1 cup coffee with sugar and cream

Lunch: 1 ham sandwich, 1 soft drink, 1 piece of pie

Dinner: Spaghetti and meat balls, mixed green salad with French dressing, French bread and 1 square butter, French pastry, coffee with sugar and cream.

The wise individual looks to the food he ingests as the major source of vitamins, minerals, and foodstuffs. Vitamin supplements taken in proper balance are acceptable, but they should not and cannot replace proper diet. When diet is planned around the four major food groups (see below) each day, additional vitamins go, for the most part, down the drain, both literally and figuratively.

The athletically inclined, who maintain a vigorous physical fitness program, *may* benefit to some extent from megavitamin therapy, using a vitamin formula containing up to ten times the amounts of vitamins listed above (with the exception of vitamin A and vitamin D). If you do so, it is important to keep in mind that definitive needs under such conditions are still being determined. It is basic that you lean on diet, not pills or capsules, for proper nutrition.

Minerals

Often forgotten in the neonlike attention created by vitamins are the mineral elements: calcium, chlorine, cobalt, copper, fluorine, iodine, iron, magnesium, manganese, potassium, phosphorus, sodium, sulfur, and zinc. A

MINERALS*

How Much Is Recommended of Key Minerals	Why Each Is Needed	Some Good Food Sources
Iron Infants 15 mg. 1-4 years 10 Over 4 18 P and L** 18	An essential part of hemoglobin, the protein substance which enables red cells to carry oxygen throughout the body. It is also part of certain important enzymes.	Liver, milk shake, fortified cereal
Calcium Infants 0.6 g. 1-4 years 0.8 Over 4 1.0 P and L 1.3	To help build strong bones and teeth. Also required for activity of nerve and muscle cells, including the heart, and for normal blood clotting.	Milk shake, ice cream, cheeseburger
Phosphorus Infants 0.5 g. 1-4 years 0.8 Over 4 1.0 P and L 1.3	Plays an essential role in the building and maintaining of strong teeth and bones, in the quick release of energy, in muscle contraction, and in nerve function.	Milk, tuna, ice cream, beef, fortified cereal
Iodine Infants 45 mcg. 1-4 years 70 Over 4 150 P and L 150	Forms an integral part of hormones produced by the thyroid gland, which is involved in the regulation of cell metabolism.	Tuna, fried clams, seafoods, iodized salt
Copper Infants 0.6 mg. 1-4 years 1.0 Over 4 2.0 P and L 2.0	Is present in many organs, including the brain, liver, heart, and kidneys. It occurs as part of important proteins, including certain enzymes involved in brain and red cell function. Also needed for making red blood cells.	Oranges, raisins, hot chocolate, nuts, mushrooms

* Vitamin Information Bureau, Inc., 664 N. Michigan Avenue, Chicago, Illinois. Reprinted with permission.

**Pregnancy and Lactation.

How Much Is Recommended of Key Minerals	Why Each Is Needed	Some Good Food Sources
Magnesium Infants 70 mg. 1-4 years 200 Over 4 400 P and L* 450	Is an important constituent of all soft tissues and bones. It helps trigger many vital enzyme reactions in humans.	French fries, corn, beef, fortified cereal
Zinc Infants 5 mg. 1-4 years 8 Over 4 15 P and L 15	Zinc appears essential for normal skeletal growth and tissue repair, and is a constituent of several important hormones, including insulin.	Milk, seafoods, eggs, beef, fortified cereal.
Chromium, Cobalt, Manganese, Molybdenum, Selenium, Fluorine Need of these substances in human nutrition established, but levels not yet determined.	Cobalt is an integral part of the vitamin B_{12} molecule. Fluorine makes teeth harder. The others are needed in a wide variety of normal body functions.	Fortified cereal, cheeseburger, beef, oranges, strawberries

*Pregnancy and Lactation.

great deal has been written about salt (sodium chloride) because of its abundance in the body and its relationship to heart disease. The role of cobalt in the formation of blood has been known for some time. The relationship of fluorine to dental cavities, potassium to cellular function, iodine to thyroid function, iron in blood-building, zinc to normal growth, and sulfur as a constituent of certain proteins (amino acids), hormones, vitamins, and enzymes is also rather common knowledge.

A number of other trace elements are present in the human body, some of which may prove indispensable, others fortuitous. Among these are aluminum, arsenic, barium, boron, bromine, cesium, lead, lithium, rubidium, silicon, strontium, tin, and titanium. Lithium has more recently come into usage in the treatment of certain mental disorders in which depression is common, but it has toxic properties and should be administered only under the supervision of a physician.

The same can be said of most minerals. You should not experiment with large doses of any mineral, as you almost certainly do more harm than good. The amounts present in many vitamin preparations are harmless and pose no threat to health, to say the least. As one pundit put it, vitamin preparations containing minerals are a "little junkier and a little heavier, but of very questionably increased efficacy." Proper diet ensures adequate mineral intake, and the following chart gives pertinent facts, RDAs, and the chief dietary sources of the minerals known to be most important to the body machine.

Protein

The solid structure of the body, other than bone, is predominantly protein, which accounts for about 20 percent of the body weight of an adult. Protein is unique in that it is the only foodstuff which can build, repair, and maintain all of the body's organs, blood cells, and tissues. Muscle and nervous tissue, as well as viscera and glands, are the principal sites where it occurs. The amino acids, of which twenty-four are known, are the basic building blocks, or protein units, from which new tissue—thousands of different proteins—is manufactured. Nine of these "bricks," or building units, cannot be manufactured by the body and must be supplied by the diet—the so-called essential amino acids. Thus it is possible for a diet to contain plentiful quantities of protein which, if of poor quality (not containing all these essential building blocks), still does not provide adequate nutrition.

Like all body constituents protein is used up and must continually be replaced. *How much* protein you need depends upon your size and on whether or not growth has been completed. Thus children require more protein, pound for pound, than do adults, and infants more than children. Pregnant and nursing women also have increased requirements in that they are feeding two or more persons. Also certain proteins are more "complete" than others, that is they contain all of the amino acids, in proportions closely resembling human tissue, and thus meet protein requirements with lesser amounts. Proteins from animal sources—beef, fowl, fish, and diary products—are superior to the protein in beans and cereal, for example, and you can meet your requirements with lesser amounts of the former. It is more desirable, however, that requirements be met from a variety of different sources.

Dr. Jean Mayer, prominent Harvard nutritionist, aptly points out that by combining different foods, each of which may be rich in different groups of amino acids, one may meet protein requirements most adequately and most economically. For example, cereals are commonly low in the amino acid lysine, while milk is rich in it; thus pouring milk on one's cereal manufactures a complete protein at the table. Similar situations occur with Italian

APPROXIMATE DAILY REQUIREMENTS FOR CALORIES,[1] PROTEIN, AND WATER*

Age in Years	Calories[2]		Protein	Water	
	Per Kg.	Per Lb.	Gm./Kg.[3]	Ml./Kg.	Oz./Lb.
Infancy[4]	110	50	3.5-2.0	150	2¼
1-3	100	45	2.5-2.0	125	2
4-6	90	41	3.0	100	1½
7-9	80	36	2.8	75	1.0+
10-12	70	32	2.0	75	1.0+
13-15	60	27	1.7	50	¾
16-19	50	23	1.5+	50	¾
Adult	40	18	0.8	50	¾

[1]Calorie = large calorie = 1 kcal = 1 cal (a calorie is a unit of heat measurement).

[2]At least 10 percent variation.

[3]To convert gm./kg. to gm./lb., divide by 2 and subtract 10 percent of the quotient. Thus 4 gm./kg. is equivalent to 1.8 gm./lb.

[4]First weeks lower; first 6 months relatively higher than last 6 months.

Equivalents: 1 gm. = 1 gram = c. 1/455 of a pound
1 kg. = 1000 gms. = c. 2.22 pounds
1 ml. = 1 milliliter = c. 1/1000 of a quart

* Adapted with permission from V.C. Vaughan and R.J. McKay, Jr., *Nelson Textbook of Pediatrics, Tenth Edition,* (Philadelphia: Saunders, 1975), p. 148.

meat sauce (low in sulfur-containing amino acids) and spaghetti made with wheat flour (rich in this essential); or with Chinese rice supplemented with beans and small amounts of meat. If you carefully select your day's menu from the basic food groups (see Appendix), you encounter no difficulty in securing this balance and variety.

The recommended daily dietary allowance of protein for an adult male is fifty-six grams (two ounces), and for an adult, nonpregnant, nonnursing female, forty-six grams (1.6 ounces). In very active persons these amounts increase proportionately.

While you may become somewhat of a dietitian by calculating the amounts of protein (as well as other foodstuffs) in your diet, such gymnastics are unnecessary if you adhere to basic requirements. It is worthwhile to realize, however, that you do not need to ingest large quantities of protein (in fact, it may be harmful) to obtain your RDA. For example, one cup of milk contains nine grams of protein, and an ounce of ground beef seven grams, an egg six, and a tablespoon of peanut butter four grams.* Two cups of milk supply about 40 percent of a woman's RDA, an added egg and three ounces of meat supply all her daily protein needs. A table showing the approximate daily requirements of protein in different age groups is shown here.

Carbohydrates

The caloric needs of the body are met chiefly by carbohydrates, which constitute the bulk of the diet. Only about 1 percent of the body weight is derived from carbohydrates stored as glycogen, mainly in the liver and muscles.

Glucose is a simple form of carbohydrate to which even complex sugars and starches must be reduced before they can be utilized by the body as fuel. Such complex carbohydrates are split at various stages in the body, beginning with the saliva, and continuing in the small intestine, into ever simpler forms, of which glucose is the chief one.

Although some glucose may be burned directly as soon as it is absorbed, especially by the brain and heart, most absorbed sugar is stored as glycogen in the liver. The combustion of glucose is an exceedingly involved process involving numerous hormones, chiefly insulin, and a number of vitamins, notably of the B-complex group. Carbohydrates which are neither burned nor stored as glycogen are converted to fat, an important consideration when dealing with the problem of overweight.

Carbodydrate requirements are such as to supply from 25 to 55 percent of the caloric intake. All too commonly, in societies such as ours, they supply closer to 50 percent of the calories.

Common sources include milk, cereals, fruits, table sugar, syrups, starches, and vegetables. There is good evidence that we ingest far too much of our carbohydrates in the simple form (sugar, syrups, and other refined sweets), as opposed to complex starches such as are found in cereal and certain breads. More is said about this later.

It is exceedingly difficult to take in too little carbohydrates unless the protein intake is less than 15 percent of the total calories, or unless starvation is present. The great anathema of our time in industrialized countries is a superfluity of carbohydrates, as it is with fat.

*Many good diet books list the protein content of most foods. The real student of nutrition should consult one of these sources.

Fats

Body fat serves a number of functions, such as being a reservoir of energy; a physical protection for vessels, nerves, and organs; insulation against cold temperatures; and a part of the structure of body tissues, cell membranes, and nuclei. It ideally constitutes no more than 15 percent of the body weight of an adult male and some 18 to 20 percent of the body weight of an adult female. Dietary fat serves as a vehicle for absorption of vitamins A, D, E, and K; provides appetite appeal and is an aid to satiety; has a protein-sparing action; and is a source of certain essential fatty acids (linoleic) which the body cannot manufacture.

Dietary fats or, more accurately, fatty substances (lipids) occur as simple lipids, compound lipids, and derived lipids.

Simple lipids are combinations of fatty acids (simple C-H chains with an acid radical) and alcohols. They constitute most of both body and dietary fat. Triglycerides (TG) are the most common of these.

Compound lipids are more complex combinations of fatty acids, alcohols, and radicals containing nitrogen, phosphorus, sugar, sulfur, or N-H radicals (amino groups). Lecithin is the best known of this group.

Derived lipids from the two preceding groups include cholesterol, well known even in lay circles, and the fatty acids (saturated and unsaturated). *Linoleic* acid is a fatty acid which cannot be manufactured by the body and must therefore be obtained from the diet.

Deficiencies of fat in the diet are, again, a rarity in industrialized countries. Excesses of fat lead to obesity and, in susceptible persons, play a role in atheromatosis, the process which plugs up arteries and leads to strokes and heart attacks.

Fat intake in this country averages 35 percent of the calories, and in some obese persons 40 percent or more. Such an intake is in excess of requirements, as populations which ingest only 10 to 15 percent of their calories as fat give no indication of nutritional problems resulting therefrom. Because of its essentiality linoleic acid should represent 1 to 2 percent of the caloric intake.

Ready sources of fat include milk, butter, egg yolk (pure cholestrol), lard, bacon, meat, fish, cheese, nuts, and vegetable oils. Dairy products and red meats (beef, pork, mutton, etc.) are especially high in saturated fats and cholesterol and triglycerides, all of which have been implicated in one way or another in our modern epidemic, coronary heart disease.

The Balanced Diet

The balanced diet is the correct answer to proper (qualitative) nutrition. Since no single food contains all the substances necessary for proper growth, nutrition, and tissue repair, balance means the inclusion of a sufficient variety of foods in the diet to ensure that all such requirements of vitamins, minerals, and major foodstuffs are met. In order to facilitate proper meal planning, foods as a whole are divided into four major groups, each of which is an especially good source of certain nutrients, and which, when used in conjunction with the other groups, guarantees a complete diet. A fifth "extra food" group is commonly included since it is often difficult to prepare a meal without such items.

By including at least one food from each of these groups in each of three meals during the day, one ensures good nutrition (see appendix).

Dietary Supplements

What about those vitamins, natural foods, and protein supplements that are flashed at the customer by the health-food industry? It simply cannot be substantiated, on a scientific basis, that most such items do what they are cracked up to do, *if* you are consuming a balanced diet day in and day out. If, however, as is so often the case, you subsist on coffee and doughnuts for breakfast, a martini and a salad with liverwurst for lunch, and an incomplete evening meal, however dressed up it may be, you just may be missing out on any number of nutrient materials essential to a sense of well-being.

In our hurried and harried society, such is not uncommonly the case, and it may explain why so many persons seem to feel better when they utilize dietary supplements. Dietary supplements should *never* be accepted as the answer to your fatigue problem until you have instituted and stuck with a well-balanced diet over a period of weeks or months. In other words they should never be a "first line of defense." If you have tried a good diet for an adequate length of time and, because of unusual stress or physical activity, still feel supplements deserve a trial, no harm can come of it if you remember the guidelines and safeguards. Summarily they are:

1. Vitamins: Do not exceed the RDA for vitamins A and D. They can be toxic in huge doses. For other vitamins select a formula which approximates that given on page 114. Unless taken at a physician's suggestion, avoid huge doses of C and E (over 1000 mgs. of vitamin C or 60 mgs. of E per day).
2. Minerals: Excesses of minerals are to be avoided. Utilize RDAs unless taken under supervision of a physician.
3. Protein supplements: Two or three tablespoonfuls in milk, once or twice daily (or two tablets three times a day), are acceptable in the well person, or if otherwise prescribed by a physician.
4. Bulk: Extra whole bran, one or two tablespoons over cereal in A.M., is quite acceptable.
5. Yeast tablets: Essentially harmless. Of questionable benefit if diet is well-rounded.

Remember! When you have to rely on dietary supplements to meet your nutritional requirements, you are admitting failure to consume a proper diet. Thus in a very real sense, the health-food industry does not supply a need. It supplements a failure.

The Prudent Diet

Because of the prevalence of cardiovascular disease (heart attacks, strokes, kidney disease) in this and other highly industrialized countries, many heart specialists are recommending a so-called prudent diet. Fatigue is a common sequel of cardiovascular disorders, and the prudent diet may be incorporated into your dietary program with no risk whatever to compromising its nutrient quality. There is also a lessening of the increased cardiovascular risk associated with the regular all-American diet. In older individuals (forty or beyond), and especially in those in which there is a strong family history of premature cardiovascular disease (heart attacks or strokes in persons under fifty), or in those with mild hypertension or obesity, such a diet is particularly beneficial. Inasmuch as fatigue commonly accompanies even mild hypertension, any measure which combats hypertension (for example, low salt diet) also combats fatigue.

Basically the prudent diet consists of the following measures:

1. Restrict sodium (salt).
2. Avoid excesses of simple refined sugars.
3. Increase usage of complex sugars and starches.
4. Restrict cholesterol intake.
5. Restrict saturated fat intake by substituting unsaturated fats whenever possible.
6. Restrict total fat intake to supply 30 percent or less of the calories.

Sodium is an element found in most common foods, usually in combination with chlorine to form sodium chloride, or table salt. Although the body needs a certain amount of sodium every day, the amount required is far less than that consumed by most people in food and drink. Even if all added salt is eliminated from the diet, a normal diet provides enough sodium to meet the MDR (minimal daily requirements).

Excesses of sodium are probably a potent factor in high blood pressure, and in diseases of the heart and blood vessels, for excess sodium causes the body to retain excess water. Such retention stresses important body functions.

Various degrees of dietary sodium restriction may be utilized, but for ordinary preventive purposes, extremes of restriction are unnecessary, and the following measures suffice:

1. Avoid use of salt in cooking or at the table.
2. Use the following only to fulfill dietary requirements: salted margarines and spreads, canned vegetables and soups, milk and milk products, certain mayonnaise and regular commercial dressings (check label for added salt); ham, bacon, sausage, and frankfurters and luncheon meats; processed fish; breads and rolls with salt topping; salted popcorn, potato chips, corn chips, pretzels, etc.; brine-preserved foods such as pickles and kraut; regular peanut butter. Note: many of the above foods may be obtained at special food stores, or in some grocery stores, with *low-salt* content (check labels).

3. Use only unsalted margarine as a spread.

Simple Sugars. Simple sugars (present in jams and jellies and candies) and *refined sugars* (table sugar) should be used as sparingly as possible (in just enough quantity to afford palatability). Sugar substitutes (for sweetening coffee, tea, etc.) are acceptable. The soda pop, the ice cream cone, the candy bar, the piece of pastry, the heaps of sugar used at the table, should become second instead of first nature, and such restrictions should be introduced early in life.

Complex Sugars and Starches. Breads, cereals, and brans supply essential bulk to the diet and shorten the emptying time of the gut. This action may lessen the likelihood of such ailments as cancer and diverticulosis of the colon, and may have a lowering effect on serum cholesterol and triglycerides, which in turn has a salutary effect on the risk of coronary heart disease.

Cholesterol. Cholesterol is a waxy derivative of true fats and is found in certain quantities in all animal tissue. Although the body manufactures a large portion of its cholesterol, a respectable amount is derived from the diet. In the United States and other countries where coronary heart disease is rampant, high cholesterol intake is the rule. It is possible to lower blood cholesterol levels by restricting its intake in the diet, although the exact effect of such lowering is the subject of much debate. When all facets of the problem are considered, however, it seems desirable to modify the cholesterol intake by substituting low-cholesterol foods for high-cholesterol ones whenever possible. Although strict diets may be built around cholesterol, the prudent dieter need only keep in mind which categories of food contain high quantities of cholesterol, and which contain low, and substitute whenever possible the latter for the former.

Saturated Fat. Saturated fat is fat which is solid at room temperature—lard, bacon fat, the fat visible on steak, roast beef, and pork—while unsaturated fat is liquid at room temperature—vegetable fats. The degree of saturation of a carbon chain with hydrogen atoms accounts for the difference, saturated fats having no room left for additional hydrogen atoms. Saturated fat intake is linked to cholesterol levels, with high intake associated with high cholesterol levels, and in turn with increased risk of heart attack. Again the prudent dieter need only be aware of foods rich in saturated fats, as opposed to those rich in unsaturated fats, and take at least one-third to one-half your total fat in unsaturated form. The following lists are aids.

Ideally no more than *30 percent of total calories* should be ingested *as fat*. Again in highly industrialized countries where heart attacks are common, 35 to 40 percent, or more, of the calories come from fat. While it is possible to calculate the daily intake of fat with the aid of tables listing fat content of the various foods, it is far easier to utilize aids in control of fat intake, cholesterol intake, and saturated fat/unsaturated fat ratio such as those available from your national or local heart association.

A variety of excellent pamphlets and booklets on the prudent diet are available from the American Heart Association, with headquarters at 7320 Greenville Avenue, Dallas, Texas. In this regard, the AHA also publishes an

FOODS HIGH IN CHOLESTEROL*

1. Dairy products:

   Egg yolk or foods containing egg yolk, such as egg noodles; some cake, pancake, and waffle mixes; some canned soups; mayonnaise and some creamy salad dressings; ice cream; many bakery products made with egg yolk.

   Butter and foods containing butterfat, such as milk (other than skim), cream; cheese made from cream or whole milk (American, Swiss); ice cream and most sherberts; many bakery products made with butter.

2. Animal tissues:

   Visible fat on bacon, pork, chicken, beef (steak and roast beef), sausage, veal, lamb.

   Lard

   Organ meats – giblets, liver, kidney, sweet breads, brains, and most packaged sandwich meats and Vienna sausage.

   Shellfish – claims, shrimp, oysters

FOODS RICH IN SATURATED FAT*

1. Foods high in cholesterol (above).

2. Some margarines, solid shortenings, chocolate, coconut, and coconut oil.

3. Don't forget foods prepared with any of the above. READ THE LABELS!

* Excerpted from *The Low Fat, Low Cholesterol Diet,* by Virginia Dobbin, Helen Gofman, *et al.* Copyright 1951 by Doubleday & Company, Inc. Reprinted by permission of the publisher.

SOME COMMON FOODS LOW IN CHOLESTEROL OR SATURATED FAT*

1. Vegetables – especially fresh; and fats of vegetable origin such as margarines and vegetable oils (cottonseed, soybean, corn, peanut, palm, olive). Chocolate, avocados, hydrogenated peanut oil as in most peanut butter, and coconut are exceptions, being high in saturated fat.
2. Fruits – especially fresh.
3. Certain dairy products such as skim milk, some buttermilk, dry cottage cheese, some sherbets.
4. Lean meat – especially some fish (halibut, whitefish, haddock); chicken and turkey in limited quantity. (Most red meats – beef, pork, mutton – are high in cholesterol and saturated fat.)
5. Dry cereals.
6. Most nuts – pecans, walnuts, almonds, peanuts, filberts.
7. Soda crackers.
8. Olives.
9. Spaghetti and macaroni.
10. Rice and tapioca.
11. Special desserts such as Jell-o, angel-food cake.
12. Miscellany such as relishes, pickles, tomato catsup, hard candy, jams, jellies, molasses, vinegar, ginger ale, yeast bread.

excellent cookbook,* rife with recipes that convert a potentially bland diet into a highly palatable one. There are, in fact, any number of good cookbooks available to help the serious-minded, prudent dieter. A few are listed here:

Virginia Dobbins, Helen Gofman, *et al., The Low Fat, Low Cholesterol Diet* (New York: Doubleday, 1951).

*Ruth Eschleman and Mary Winston, *The American Heart Association Cookbook* (New York: McKay, 1973). Paperback by Ballantine Books, New York, 1976.

Jeanne Jones, *Diet for a Happy Heart* (San Francisco: 101 Productions, 1975).

Helen Cassidy Page and John Speer Schroeder, M.D., *The Whole Family Low Cholesterol Cookbook* (New York: Grosset & Dunlap, 1976).

CHAPTER 10

Our Nutritional Dilemma

A good friend of mine utilizes the following dietary supplements, in which all meals are high protein, moderate fat, low carbohydrate, with no sugar, no coffee, and only weak tea allowed:

*Breakfast Vitamin C, .500 mg.
Multiple vitamin
Vitamin E, 400 Units

Niacin, 100 mg.
Glutamic acid, 500 mg.
Vitamin B-complex

"Cocktail" (½ glass orange juice, ½ glass water, 1 tablespoon full soya powder, 1 tablespoon full yeast, 1 tablespoon full lecithin, 1 tablespoon wheat germ oil, salt)

Mid-morning Niacin, 100 mg.
Glutamic acid, 500 mg.
12 yeast tablets
B-complex

Lunch 400 units vitamin E

Niacin, 100 mg.
B-complex
Glutamic acid, 500 mg.
Vitamin C

*High-protein breakfasts have more recently been connected with a sense of well-being, while fatigue has been associated with low-protein intake at the first meal.

Mid-afternoon B-complex

Niacin, 100 mg.
Glutamic acid, 500 mg.
12 desiccated liver tablets

Late afternoon	Soya beans, or nuts with diet drink
Dinner	"Dessert" 2 tablespoons yeast powder in one glass milk sweetened with saccharin
Bedtime	Light snack (peanut butter and crackers, cheese, apple, meat, hard-boiled egg, etc.)

Note: Carbohydrate intake is increased some with increased physical activity.

A megavitamin product of the new nutrition, he and millions like him account for a sizable hunk of the $121 billion spent each year on health care in America. Yet life expectancy remains essentially unchanged. Why? Because Americans as a whole still suffer from malnutrition—the malnutrition of too much. Too much sugar, too much fat, too much salt, too many calories. For example, a diet low in salt is unquestionably beneficial to high blood pressure. Yet in the United States we consume more than ten pounds of salt per person per year—and one adult in seven has high blood pressure. Removing the salt shaker from the table helps, but it is not enough; too much of our salt is in processed foods, including baby foods as a starter. Our diets, unfortunately and unscientifically, are the products of flavor engineering, and fast foods have become popular national meals.

Physician monitorings of a major TV channel for a single week in 1970 revealed only 5 percent of total TV time to be devoted to health information; 90 percent of this time was considered inaccurate or misleading.

But this is not all our problem. Although more than fifty nutrients are now recognized as being essential to full health, the list continues to grow. Primitive man was no scientist, but his diet—roots and shoots, bugs and berries, rodents and reptiles—was nutritionally correct.

Even in the more primitive civilizations of today, diets that are substandard to the best of our dietitians still support life longer and more actively than those of which the average American avails himself. The villagers of Vilcabamba, living on a high-starch, low-protein, "calorically inadequate" fare, boast active lives well into their nineties and produce centenarians at a rate 300 to our one. The Tarahawara Indians, on 1,500 calories per day derived chiefly from corn products and beans, run one hundred miles a day in pursuit of a wooden ball over rocky, hilly terrain. Pure vegetarians from many populations of the world maintain seemingly excellent health.

What does all this mean? It means that, over the centuries, modern man has "cultured" himself into a nutritional corner. It means that there is still much to be learned about nutrition, and that possibly the best place to learn it is from our predecessors who lived close to the good earth, and from those who still do.

PART THREE

The Management of Mental Fatigue

CHAPTER 11

Management Techniques

Mental fatigue is a state which often lies next door to sleep. A natural question arises when you are combatting mental fatigue: should you sleep or should you try to do something else? If you are faced with a rest deficit—obviously behind on your rest—then sleep is the answer. Quite often I find that if I have had a night riddled with phone calls which have punctuated my sleep, mental endeavors (reading, writing, chart work) are best helped if I take a short snooze on my office couch during the noon break. Unless a sleep deficit exists, however, the answer to mental fatigue is *stimulating diversion*. Such diversion implies engagement in a different type of activity than the one causing mental fatigue. For example, if you are a secretary, you would most likely not be stimulated by typing as a diversionary activity.

Use of Stimuli

Mental stimulation may also counter mental fatigue. The reading of an interesting and exciting book, for example, may have such an effect; so also talk sessions in the presence of an interesting discussant of a lively topic; or playing certain games, or solving puzzles, or writing on an interesting subject. But such ploys cannot hope to achieve the same overall results as good exercise programs. The physiologic basis is simply not the same.

Emotional stimulation certainly combats mental fatigue, but again, it must have unusual content to even approach the effects of exercise. Stimulating radio or TV programs may fall into this category. Debates or conversations or discussions on partisan issues may fill the bill. Certain types of printed material also tickles the adrenals, especially if argumentative in nature and running contrary to the beliefs of the reader.

Summarily, then, mental fatigue is best and most naturally counteracted by the stimulatory effect of the right amount and kind and duration of physical activity. As you shall see, there is some such activity available to practically everyone. Nowadays, with leisure time more plentiful and employers more efficiency-conscious, it is more and more easy for you to plan some such activity at some time during the day. Mental and emotional stimulatory aids are, at best, poor substitutes for physical activity in warding off mental fatigue.

Avoidance of Monotony

Monotonous repetition of an act, whether on a minute-to-minute or hour-to-hour basis (as in hemstitching), or on a day-to-day basis (as repeating the same housekeeping chores), or even a year-to-year basis (as practicing pediatrics), is the sine qua non for production of mental fatigue. Sameness, stereotyped activity, repetition carried on so long that the act, whatever it is, can be performed without serious challenge of the mental processes, almost guarantees mental fatigue. Mary, for example, had a job doing stitching on a machine in a clothing factory. She became so adept at it that she could almost perform the task in her sleep. She also developed chronic fatigue. She requested a trial in the sales department, where she became quite successful, and the fatigue disappeared.

Dr. Helen was an insurance physician who performed routine physical exams on insurance applicants. After a time the procedure became so routine that the doctor was tired throughout her working day (but felt strangely alive again after it was over). She sought and got a job with an industrial plant as plant physician; here the work was quite varied, new, and stimulating, and her daytime fatigue disappeared. These examples illustrate how it is possible to strike at the root of the problem of mental fatigue—abolish repetitiveness, sameness, and monotony. Where it is possible to do this, purely mental fatigue almost always disappears. Often, however, it is not possible to be so drastic in your approach to the problem. In such instances you must rely on other techniques, notably diversion, innovation, and the carrot-on-the-stick approach.

Diversionary Tactics

A diversion is any tactic, maneuver, or ploy—mental or physical, brief or prolonged—which is injected into a routinized pattern of occupation, avocation, or existence, in order to give fresh content to life and break up monotony. It obviously should be pleasant and must adapt to restrictions of time, money, and circumstances.

The most time-honored diversionary tactic is the coffee break, and employees have been known to quit good jobs because it was missing. It has become an institution in itself. However, as has been pointed out, there are better ways of achieving the same results.

I have already alluded to the exercise break, and say a great deal more about exercise later. To achieve their purpose, exercise breaks ordinarily require more time than coffee breaks, as well as special facilities and equipment. Also, a supervisor of such activity is desirable or essential in many instances. For these reasons, despite their many good points, such breaks have been slow to come into full acceptance. However, even where such breaks are not a part of company policy, the employee may, by permission, of course, convert his coffee break into a simple exercise break. If nothing more, he may spend the time ordinarily spent in sitting down while consuming coffee into a brisk walk—whether on downtown sidewalks or amongst more pastoral surroundings.

Noon breaks afford more time and an excellent spot in the day's routine for more organized activity, such as volleyball or basketball. They may also be used for individual efforts such as jogging or cycling. In a later chapter the flexibility of exercise methods becomes obvious. With a little ingenuity and planning, there are very few occupations which cannot allow for activity of some type or degree.

John, a legal typist in a large urban center, solved his problem by joining a nearby Y and utilizing its facilities at noon. Joe, also bound in by concrete and steel, solved his problem (and his associates') by being instrumental in getting a jogging track installed on the roof of his office building.

Dr. Charles kept a bicycle at a cycle shop near his office and rode around a nearby lake during the noon hour. Many a dull routine has thus been converted into an enjoyable, healthy, more productive merry-go-round. If you find yourself under similar job circumstances, no doubt with a bit of thought you can come up with your own version of what these persons did.

Thus far considered have been chiefly the midmorning, noontime, and P.M. breaks. What about varying your means of getting to and from work? Could you use a bicycle—either all the way or partway? Could you drive to the fringe of town with a cycle on a cycle rack, park, and cycle the rest of the way? Could you do the same for walking? Lots of traffic headaches can be beat in this fashion. If you have shower facilities at work, you might eventually consider jogging to work and back (even some senators are doing this nowadays).

Whenever diversion can be combined with utilitarianism (such as contributing to one's health while cutting down on transportation expense), so much the better; motivation is multiplied, as are end results.

Still other types of diversion have already been alluded to. Company game rooms (dominoes, chess, whatever) and libraries, even with limited facilities, can improve dull situations a great deal. Radios in appropriate places, TV sets in cold-drink or lounge areas, may all contribute to diversion.

Gregarious persons can team up against boredom in a variety of ways. A group of nightworkers in a factory organized an astronomy club and used their break to study the stars from a rooftop observatory. A group of dayworkers took up bird watching at a nearby lake (which, incidentally, has excellent sailing facilities). Others formed a co-op buyers' association for household items, including groceries, and held their meetings at noon two or three times a week. A group of doctors in a medical building formed a stock-and-bond club that met at noon. One very industrious bunch of refinery workers leased a field across from the plant and raised their own farm products, keeping the necessary implements in a company warehouse. The possibilities for creating diversion from dull routine are almost endless, bounded only by the imagination (or lack of it) of the person(s) involved.

Company policies toward work diversion are fast changing. Happier, more productive workers are, after all, any manager's dream. A number of top corporations in Texas and California have organized basketball and soccer teams. Others have jogging paths around their headquarters. One large Dallas-based industry sports a gym, tennis courts, and gun club, still another a belly-dancing club. A Rhode Island company opened a library and sponsors singing lessons for employees and their children. Purchases for the industrial recreation market are big business, to the tune of $3.5 billion annually. If you have an idea about diversion you can suggest to your supervisor, do it. It could win you a lot of points in a lot of ways. For professional help contact one or both of the following:

National Industrial Recreation Association
20 North Wacker Drive
Chicago, Illinois 60606

American Association of Fitness Directors in
Business and Industry
c/o President's Council on Physical
Fitness and Sports
Washington, D.C. 20201

Use of Innovations

Innovation differs from diversion in that while diversion is a turning away from your work pattern, innovation refers to changing the work pattern itself. Creativity may play a dominant role. Bill was a maintenance man on a production line for a large food-processing plant; he found his work quite boring and mentally fatiguing until he was allowed to use his mechanical genius to redesign some of the machinery for the better, improving production and reducing expense. Not only did his mental fatigue disappear, but thereafter he found the job both challenging and rewarding (he even received due recompense for his ingenuity).

Mary, who changed from hemstitching to sales in a drygoods company, is still another example of innovation. Jim was on an auto assembly line and grew tired of putting the same nuts and bolts in the same holes, as it were; he devised a rotation system which allowed him and a group of fellow workers to work on different assemblies from time to time, in rotary fashion, such that the monotony was broken up; it met the approval of his foreman and proved a boon not only to him, but to fellow workers as well. Finding a new and easier way to do a tedious task, designing new tools if needed, and developing new ideas that relate to your job all afford a challenge and a stimulus which often convert tedium and fatigue into a whole new ballgame. Moreover the contributions of such an employee are likely to be recognized by the alert employer and not go unrewarded.

The Carrot-on-the-Stick

An old cartoon has a stick, tied to the back of a donkey, projecting out beyond the donkey's face with a carrot dangling from its tip just out of reach of the donkey's nose. In his effort to get to the carrot, the animal propels the cart which he is pulling with a great deal of verve. In similar fashion, the racing greyhound can be spurred on to greater heights if he is chasing a rabbit. And so it is with the worker faced with a monotonous task, with the endless "pulling of the cart," if you will. Such a person, trodding monotonously along, finds renewed vigor and inspiration if, at a break period, or at the end of the day, or at the end of a year for that matter, a "carrot" awaits him in the form of a pleasure or an avocation or a reward to which he can look ahead. Such company-supplied "carrots" as coffee breaks and noon breaks have already been considered. You can supply some "carrots" of your own. If John is avocationally a woodworker, for example, but needs tools to fully equip his home shop, he can endure a lot of monotony in his regular work if, in the process, he is aware that he is saving up funds to buy that equipment. Once the shop is complete, he may even turn an avocation into a paying vocation. So the shop is the "carrot" for which John pulls his cart.

Denise is an artist who attends night painting classes after work three times a week. She is also converting an attic room into a studio. Her job as a telephone operator is quite monotonous, but she looks forward during the day to her artwork in the evening and sets aside some of each two weeks' pay toward the finishing of her studio. Mary's art is the "carrot" that enables her to pull her "cart." And so on.

Everyone needs a carrot-on-a-stick. Too many Joes and Janes go through life, or attempt to do so, with nothing challenging, nothing stimulating, nothing to look forward to, nothing to work toward; content, or rather malcontent, to trudge along with everything behind them and nothing before. I once had a nurse who worked diligently and faithfully for many a year, despite handicaps, in order to send two children to college. I doubt seriously if she would have endured the monotony and drudgery of numerous years of sameness had it not been for the "carrot"—seeing her children receive a college degree. That one brief moment of time made her long years of fatigue endurable and worth the while.

It is obvious that the carrot-on-the-stick policy applies also to lifetime goals (which are considered in the next chapter), and to avocations. Many an avocation has become a vocation. And there is no better carrot than a stimulating avocation. Consider the fireman who used his time sitting around the station to study electronics, developed TV repair as a hobby he pursued when off duty, and finally quit his firefighting to open his own TV repair shop. Or the school teacher who was a devoted bass fisherman that spent every off hour on a lake and became so adept at his avocation and fell so in love with the outdoors, that it was inevitable that he quit teaching and become a professional guide. Or the traveling salesman who carried a camera with him everywhere he went. He had such a nose for the unusual and a quickness with the lens that he was able to sell much of his material to various news media for a nice profit.

Other than primary goals, avocations are the most effective "carrots" ever devised. Again, if you are faced with the drudgery-fatigue problem and don't have a "carrot," get one, by all means. And you need not stop with only one. Pursue a physical avocation (jogging, gardening, boating) for health and a mental one (stamp collecting, a new line of endeavor in night school or by correspondence) for profit. The possibilities are endless. All you have to do is start looking. Over the long haul, it may change your entire life; over the short haul, it can convert that monotonous routine of yours into a welcome necessity.

PART FOUR

The Management of Chronic Emotional Fatigue

As stated at the beginning, the emotional type of chronic fatigue is by far the most common. As also pointed out no one type of fatigue (physical, mental, or emotional) exists alone. Thus the principles for combatting physical and mental fatigue are also involved in the management of emotional fatigue. The diet must be proper and adequate. Rest must be regular and of sufficient duration. Diversions and avocations are just as important to the relief of emotional fatigue as they are to relief of mental fatigue, perhaps moreso, but for different reasons.

Management of chronic emotional fatigue revolves, basically, around relief of stress and strain, with special attention to the following areas as pointed out by Drs. Robert S. Eliot and Alan D. Forker* of the University of Nebraska Medical Center: (1) establishment of priorities; (2) identifying objective, realistic, and obtainable goals; (3) attempting behavior modification of type-A personality; (4) reducing the frequency of stressful life-change events; (5) teaching the daily technique of the relaxation response; (6) aerobic physical exercise; (7) group therapy. It is items such as these which, therefore, concern us in the pages just ahead.

*R.S. Eliot, M.D. and A.D. Forker, M.D., "Emotional Stress and Cardiac Disease," *Journal of the American Medical Association*, 236 (1976): 2325-2326. By permission.

CHAPTER 12

Depression: A Special Consideration

Depression cannot be dismissed lightly in any consideration of fatigue. According to one survey, over 50 percent of Americans report feeling depressed at one time or another. 15 percent of American adults may be seriously depressed. The National Association for Mental Health has indicated that depression is now pushing schizophrenia as the top-ranking mental-health problem. It is likely that no one escapes the clutches of depression at some time in life; it is known to occur even in infancy, and the increasing incidence of suicides in adolescence (the second leading cause of death in this age group) attests to its prevalence in the formative years. Depression is inextricably involved in our rapidly ascending rates of divorce and crime.

What Is Depression?

Depression is a mood disturbance characterized by dejection, feelings of despair or hopelessness, and a negative outlook on life in general. No concise definition is available, but as Professor of Psychiatry Hugh Storrow of the University of Kentucky College of Medicine has pointed out, the following characteristics are generally present:*

1. There is a persistent mood of sadness, apathy, or loneliness.
2. There are convictions of hopelessness and pessimism about ever feeling better, even though the involved person recognizes such convictions are illogical.
3. The depressed person tends to blame himself for his problems and those surrounding him.
4. Wishes to escape through running away, hiding, or dying are common.
5. General levels of activity—speaking, acting, whatever—are reduced. Unproductive restlessness and agitation may occur.
6. Certain physical symptoms, such as insomnia (especially a tendency to awaken early), loss of appetite (with or without weight loss), loss of libido, and chronic fatigue are commonplace.

While the recognition of severe depression, with suicidal tendencies and overtly psychotic activity, is relatively easy, the recognition of mild to

**Depression in Medical Practice*. Edited by A.J. Enelow, Merck, Sharpe & Dohme, West Point, Pa., 1970. pp. 25-26.

moderate depression, appearing as it does behind many masks, is sometimes quite difficult and requires all the diagnostic skill of the most astute physician. Dr. Aaron Beck (Professor of Psychiatry, University of Pennsylvania) has developed a Depression Inventory (reproduced here) which is very helpful to patient and physician alike in the recognition of this very ubiquitous emotional problem. If interested you may take a self-inventory and score yourself as follows:

0-9:	Healthy mental state
10-15:	Mild depression
16-23:	Moderate depression
24 and over:	Severe depression

The Beck Depression Inventory*

A. 0 I do not feel sad.
1 I feel sad.
2 I am sad all the time and I can't snap out of it.
3 I am so sad or unhappy that I can't stand it.

B. 0 I am not particularly discouraged about the future.
1 I feel discouraged about the future.
2 I feel I have nothing to look forward to.
3 I feel that the future is hopeless and that things cannot improve.

C. 0 I do not feel like a failure.
1 I feel I have failed more than the average person.
2 As I look back on my life, all I can see is a lot of failures.
3 I feel I am a complete failure as a person.

D. 0 I get as much satisfaction out of things as I used to.
1 I don't enjoy things the way I used to.
2 I don't get real satisfaction out of anything anymore.
3 I am dissatisfied or bored with everything.

E. 0 I don't feel particularly guilty.
1 I feel guilty a good part of the time.
2 I feel quite guilty most of the time.
3 I feel guilty all of the time.

F. 0 I don't feel I am being punished.
1 I feel I may be punished.
2 I expect to be punished.
3 I feel I am being punished.

*Reproduced by permission of Aaron T. Beck, M.D., Professor of Psychiatry, University of Pennsylvania School of Medicine, Philadelphia, Pa., and *Medical Opinion*, 575 Madison Ave., New York, New York.

G. 0 I don't feel disappointed in myself.
1 I am disappointed in myself.
2 I am disgusted with myself.
3 I hate myself.

H. 0 I don't feel I am any worse than anybody else.
1 I am critical of myself for my weaknesses or mistakes.
2 I blame myself all the time for my faults.
3 I blame myself for everything bad that happens.

I. 0 I don't have any thoughts of killing myself.
1 I have thoughts of killing myself, but I would not carry them out.
2 I would like to kill myself.
3 I would kill myself if I had the chance.

J. 0 I don't cry any more than usual.
1 I cry more now than I used to.
2 I cry all the time now.
3 I used to be able to cry, but now I can't cry even though I want to.

K. 0 I am no more irritated now than I ever am.
1 I get annoyed or irritated more easily than I used to.
2 I feel irritated all the time now.
3 I don't get irritated at all by the things that used to irritate me.

L. 0 I have not lost interest in other people.
1 I am less interested in other people than I used to be.
2 I have lost most of my interest in other people and have little feeling for them.
3 I have lost all of my interest in other people and don't care about them at all.

M. 0 I make decisions about as well as I ever could.
1 I put off making decisions more than I used to.
2 I have greater difficulty in making decisions than before.
3 I can't make decisions at all anymore.

N. 0 I don't feel I look any worse than I used to.
1 I am worried that I am looking old or unattractive.
2 I feel that there are permanent changes in my appearance that make me look unattractive.
3 I believe that I look ugly.

O. 0 I can work about as well as before.
1 It takes an extra effort to get started at doing something.
2 I have to push myself very hard to do anything.
3 I can't do any work at all.

P. 0 I can sleep as well as usual.
1 I don't sleep as well as I used to.
2 I wake up one to two hours earlier than usual and find it hard to get back to sleep.
3 I wake up several hours earlier than I used to and cannot get back to sleep.

Q. 0 I don't get more tired than usual.
1 I get tired more easily than I used to.
2 I get tired from doing almost anything.
3 I am too tired to do anything.

R. 0 My appetite is no worse than usual.
1 My appetite is not as good as it used to be.
2 My appetite is much worse now.
3 I have no appetite at all anymore.

S. 0 I haven't lost much weight, if any, lately.
1 I have lost more than 5 pounds.
2 I have lost more than 10 pounds.
3 I have lost more than 15 pounds.

(I am purposely trying to lose weight by eating less. Disregard this question if answer is yes.)

T. 0 I am no more worried about my health than usual.
1 I am worried about physical problems such as aches and pains, or up-set stomach, or constipation.
2 I am very worried about physical problems, and it's hard to think of much else.
3 I am so worried about my physical problems that I cannot think about anything else.

U. 0 I have not noticed any recent change in my interest in sex.
1 I am less interested in sex than I used to be.
2 I am much less interested in sex now.
3 I have lost interest in sex completely.

While this inventory is a valuable guide in enabling you to arrive at your mental status with regard to depression, it is sometimes difficult, as with any self-examination, to be as totally objective and detached as need be. The finding of mild depression is no cause for concern unless it is a persistent, unvarying state. Moods are subject to great variation from day to day, and an inventory taken on a down day may not be the same as that on an up day. A score of fifteen or more, however, indicates that depression is very likely a significant factor in your chronic fatigue problem. And if the score is in the severe range, psychiatric help is definitely in order, is in fact urgent.

The importance of the recognition of severe depression by the chronically fatigued is that the methodology for combatting fatigue as outlined in this book is inadequate to totally supplant expert psychiatric help. Certainly if after proper institution of the measures herein recommended, a feeling of general improvement is not promptly experienced, expert psychiatric help should be sought. If at any time suicidal thoughts become frequent and overpowering, seek medical help at once! On the other hand, the individual suffering from only mild to moderate depression may find that implementation of the methods shortly to be considered is all he needs to turn the tide of his fatigue. In particular, attention should be directed to the section on physical activity. Physical activity has long been recognized as a valuable tool in the treatment of anxiety, depression, and other emotional problems.

Just as the depressed person who busies himself feels some relief from depression, at least temporarily, so does the depressed person who develops a vigorous physical activity program manufacture a superb outlet for his frustrations and hostilities, which are often part and parcel of depression. Such a program may serve as a much-needed outlet for pent-up emotions which, undischarged, multiply the seeds of depression and fatigue. More than one depressed person—overweight, mildly hypertensive, and unwilling to become involved—has, through a program of vigorous physical activity, found welcome relief for his symptoms, if not his underlying problems. Certainly any able-bodied individual in such a category, who neglects the use of this important tool, is bypassing a simple and natural outlet, the adequate use of which might well solve his entire problem and change the entire course of his life.

If chronic emotional fatigue (which is the result of chronic anxiety, which is the product of chronic stress) is to be combatted properly, it is obvious that chronic stress must be reduced. In such a consideration, let us again focus our attention upon (1) the goal, (2) the environment (and its obstacles), and (3) the subject.

CHAPTER 13

Setting Goals

Before you can seriously consider changing goal(s), it is important that you know something about setting them in the first place. Goals should fit, like a good suit of clothes. They should be comfortable to the wearer.

Unfortunately there are too many square pegs in round holes in all walks of life. A boy or girl studies medicine because a parent is a doctor, or because the parent wants the tradition continued (grandfather was one also). Little Mary winds up a piano teacher because father just knew she had the hands of a concert artist. If the long-term goal doesn't fit the subject—if he is striving for something that basically has no appeal—then the best thing that he can do is to face up to it and, where possible, make a change. The same can be said of intermediate, short-term, even immediate goals. If you find yourself feeling out of character in what you strive for, or it is to your dislike, or you'd rather be doing something else, then it's time to switch.

I have two sons, one of whom aspires to study medicine; but I have made it a point never to twist his arm in that direction. What I have emphasized, rather, is that each one do what he would rather do than anything else in the world—regardless of how known or unknown he might be, regardless of whether he makes $100 a week or $50,000 a year, regardless of whether he wears a white shirt or a blue denim one. I still think that's good advice. Never set a goal because of whimsy, or the vicarious wishes of another (to please someone else), or the enticement of making money or a name, as many, many persons do or have done. Consider the profession of medicine, since I am most familiar with it. I know a surgeon or two who should have been internists, an anesthesiologist who would have been happier as a surgeon, and any number of pediatricians who should have been just about any other kind of doctor. And I have known some doctors who shouldn't have been doctors at all. The same can be said for a large segment of just about any kind of occupation—lawyers, plumbers, bankers, whatever.

One national periodical circulated amongst doctors revealed, from a poll, that only about two thirds of the pediatricians surveyed stated they would take up pediatrics again if they had it to do over. About 20 percent of the internists were unhappily engaged, and 15 percent of the psychiatrists, and so on.

The point is: there are too many people pursuing goals for which they are, in one way or another, unsuited. And the result is stress, tension, and fatigue. It is stress, tension, and fatigue built into the life structure of that individual simply because he is training or has trained for an occupation to which he does not belong.

CHAPTER 14

Tackling Goals

The Real Biggies

Major Decisions

According to the pundits there are three major decisions which one must make in establishing a life pattern. (1) What shall I do for a livelihood? (2) Whom shall I marry? (Or *shall* I marry?) (3) Where shall I live? All major goals, in fact, revolve about and derive from these decisions. These foundational decisions are so important that enormous input should go into the between-the-ears computer before final conclusions are reached. Such decisions, once made, should for all practical purposes be irrevocable. Pragmatically this is not always possible. Exigencies arise. Circumstances change. But insofar as humanly attainable, you should be able to answer the question, "Is this the right decision?", with a resounding and unhesitating YES!

If there exists any hesitation, the slightest uncertainty, the faintest doubt, then the computer should be kept open. Reassess. Rethink. Investigate. In short, be 99.99 percent certain of your conclusion. So critically important are these foundational areas of life, that any decision regarding them should be the product of blood, sweat, and tears, as it were. They are the launching pad for the goals that follow. The importance of their due and just consideration cannot be overemphasized if stress and its by-products are to be avoided.

Trial Runs

When setting out in pursuit of a lifetime goal, it's far better to be on the right track from the outset than to try to get into another one later on. But there are many instances in which trial runs are necessary before you can really decide whether a certain pursuit is your cup of tea. For example, a high school student may think he would like to be an auto mechanic, but a month or two as an apprentice in an auto repair shop convinces him that he was wrong. Another may feel inclined to study law, but a summer job in a lawyer's office shows him the folly of his aspirations. Trial runs may save considerable stress if they are recognized as such and not pursued far beyond the point where it is obvious that one is barking up the wrong tree.

There are any number of tests—psychological and otherwise—which the young aspirant can take to help determine his strong points, his likes and dislikes, and so on. There are trained individuals who conduct such tests, some of them quite involved, to try to get you into the right starting gate. But even these leave something to be desired. A certain amount of trial and error is essential, if not inevitable, with any worthwhile undertaking. On the other hand the guy who rolls the dice and heads north if they come up snake eyes, south on a seven, east on a trey, probably is too immature to decide on a goal in the first place.

Goal Assessments

A very desirable tack, whether starting out in life or whether well along in it, is to have a time for *periodic goal assessments*. For example, you might review long-term goals annually, at, say, New Year's (but with the clearest of heads, please). Intermediate and short-term goals might be studied more often. Immediate goals can be reviewed from week to week, even day to day. I try to set aside five or ten minutes each A.M. to either mentally fix in mind, or jot down on paper, what I need to do that day and assign some order of priority to the various items. Carry out goal assessments faithfully and regularly. Maintain flexible thinking. Are there better routes? Is there a shortcut? What's new? And so on. An on-the-toes approach to goals with an open mind is the best preventive I know to weaving webs from which you cannot escape.

Goal Qualities

Various qualities, or attributes, of goals must always be considered. These include desirability, proximity, elusiveness, concreteness, complexity, realisticality, and clarity. You have looked briefly at these in Chapter 3, and they are considered in terms of the management of relieving stress in a subsequent section.

Organization of Goals

Mini- and maxigoals alike have a much better chance of being realized if you organize your approach. What this means for the long-term goal is that staging of the various steps be done as far in advance as possible, so that, as we have already pointed out, the long-term goal is broken down into intermediate goals and the intermediate goal into short-term goals. It's a lot like running an obstacle race. You may know in what general direction the finish line lies, but you must focus attention on the bog, or the hurdle, or the stretch of roadway just ahead, and take each obstacle in stride.

Organization means planning—by the year, the month, the week, even the day—using facts, knowledge, foresight, and wisdom wherever they can be gleaned. Try to have a regular, appointed time for each activity as it relates to your goal(s). One doctor who has the so-called Midas Touch operates all morning, three days a week, and runs a hospital and nursing home the other two. His afternoons, save one during which he golfs, are devoted to his patients. His noonhour, aside from the one on his afternoon off, is devoted to running or tennis, or both. And from five to six P.M. each afternoon, before making hospital rounds, he devotes to various business enterprises. His weekends are equally well-planned, as are his vacations. You might almost argue that he's too well-organized, but he has accomplished more in forty-five years than the average man in seventy.

The whole point is this: if your goals are many, and you want to save yourself a lot of stress and fatigue, plan your time and utilize it well. Not only will you operate with less anxiety and tension, thus being more efficient and accomplishing a great deal more, but you are far more likely to enjoy what you do. What's more, you'll find you have more time to devote to other goals, or diversions—whatever you like—time that is relatively free of the tension and anxiety generated by cluttered up days and weeks and years.

Another doctor never seemed to have quite enough time to accomplish all that he wanted to do. He seemed, so he said, to be always playing catch up, trying to find a spare moment to pursue some project he never seemed to have time for. He was always, he said, too tired to scrounge out more time from his already hectic day. In response to my inquiry, he stated he usually went to bed at 11 P.M. and his alarm sounded at 7 A.M., but that his nights were so interrupted by periods of insomnia (during which he pondered over the many things he never seemed to get around to) that he couldn't get up when the alarm sounded. I suggested that the next time he so awakened, he should get up and go to his study and dive into a correspondence course he had long been trying to finish.

"Make yourself get up and use that early morning time, even if it's only thirty minutes to start with." He looked at me as if I had been chewing loco weed at first, then said he might give it a try. I saw him a few weeks later.

"Say," he said, "you might like to know I've taken your advice about that night stuff. The first two or three study rounds, and the day after, were murder. But since then I've fiinished my correspondence course and got another project going. What's more, I sleep like a baby and get up when the alarm goes off. And I'm not tired any more. I even feel up to working on an evening project now. In fact, I've accomplished more in the last month than in the preceding year, I think."

This doctor was poorly organized, a classic example of stress begetting stress. What he did was to make himself get up and use some early morning time that he had previously spent in needless and fruitless anxiety. He converted worrytime into studytime, useless time into useful time. And it cured his fatigue problem, at least temporarily. With a bit of planning and organization, most of us could come up with a similar bonus. There's an old cliche: if you want something done, call a busy man. To paraphrase: if you want something done, call an organized man.

Aids and Abetments

In his pursuit of a goal, the wise man uses any source of information or wisdom he can get—libraries, books, schools (night courses, correspondence), and above all, people! The empirical wisdom of an expert may be worth more than a library full of ponderous tomes on a subject.

If your goal is to make a million dollars by the time you're forty-five (and you're twenty-five now and have a $10,000 nest egg to start with), you'd better read some pretty potent books on money-making, attend some top-notch seminars, and get to know some highly successful financiers. If your approach is one of "going to Vegas and betting on red," get set for a lot of headaches, tension, and fatigue—not to mention separation from what money you have. For every long-shot millionaire, there must be at least ten who consulted every source of information available to them along the way.

To start off in pursuit of a goal without all the help you can get (in the way of information and guidance) is akin to going elephant hunting without gun or guide. The one who does so is just asking for all kinds of stress and anxiety.

Never be too proud to admit you're dumb about a given subject, especially if you are. But don't stop there. Do something about it. Fill the void with facts and good advice. You'll most likely reach your goal, but if you don't, you'll be a lot less tired for the trying if you look before you leap. And you'll be that much more likely to succeed the next time around.

Assigning Goal Priorities

Rearrangement of priorities presupposes that some order of priority has been assigned to goals in the first place. Often this is not the case. All too often, goals move in and out of conscious thought or activity like so many ghosts, recognized poorly or not at all. The serious person, especially when confronted with chronic emotional fatigue, needs to sit down and outline his goals and assign them priorities to the best of his ability, even though it may be necessary to rearrange them the very next day.

How Do You Arrive at Priorities? You can begin by jotting down the goal categories, and then arranging them in order of their importance in your life. Following is a suggested list with which to begin, numbered in a suggested order of priority:

1. Health
2. Family
3. Vocation
4. Avocation
5. Leisure Activity

The order of priority given each category is subject to change with each individual. For example, to some persons vocational goals are more important than family goals.

Next supply subheadings to the major headings, somewhat as follows. Note that there may be overlaps between the various areas.

1. Health
   a. Annual medical checkup
   b. Diet
   c. Exercise

2. Family
   a. Financial (security)
   b. Housing
   c. Education
   d. Leisure

3. Vocation
   a. Improve work knowledge or skill
   b. Improve work conditions
   c. Shoot for raise (increase financial return)

4. Avocation
   a. Correspondence course
   b. Shop in garage

5. Leisure-time activity
   a. Exercise program
   b. Time with family
   c. Vacation

Continue to subdivide the subheadings. For example, you might jot down the following under Family:

2. Family
   a. Financial (security)
      1. Check insurance program
      2. Go over budget
   b. Housing
      1. Get estimate on home repairs
   c. Education
      1. Start college savings fund for kids
      2. Check on trust for kids
   d. Leisure
      1. Possible family boat (?)
      2. Possible weekend retreat (?)

Next divide the subheadings into groups according to their immediacy (immediate, short-term, intermediate, or long-term goal), as in the following chart:

Order of Importance ↓	Goals	Immediate (Today) (Next Week)	Short-term (Next 6 Months to 1 Year)	Inter-mediate (6 Months to 5 Years)	Long-term (Over 5 Years)
	Health	Checkup Diet			
	Finances & Security	Get with broker			Net worth $100G
	Family		Kids/private school funds House re-modeled	New house Family boat	
	Vocation	Early to work Talk/boss	Get raise?		
	Avocation	Regular PE program	Start corre-spondence course		

When properly arranged, there should be a natural "flow" of immediate goals toward short-term ones, short-term toward intermediate, and intermediate toward long-term. Furthermore, the goals in one category should complement the goals in another. Thus, a financial goal (long-term) of $100,000 net worth is aided and abetted by a short-term goal of getting a raise, and quite possibly by the short-term goal of starting a correspondence course. The immediate goal of checking up on your health status is basic to all goals, since without good health other goals lose a great deal of their worth, and since good health is vital to carrying out projects.

By and large, such a chart should indicate roughly, at a glance, your goals in order of importance from top toward bottom, that is, arranged in order of decreasing importance from the top down, and the order in which your goals should be accomplished over the long haul (reading from left to right). As the months and years pass, immediate goals should fuse into short-term goals, and short-term into intermediate, and so on. For example, the short-term goal of remodeling the house will aid and abet its sale toward purchase of a new house (intermediate goal). Thus the flow of activity should be from left to right on the chart, and it is to immediate and short-term priorities that one can assign numbers and set aside certain time(s) in which nothing shall interfere with the carrying out of that priority. To do this, it is necessary to break down (subdivide) even further such subheadings as shown on the preceding page. Again consider two or three immediate goals.

Goals	**Immediate**
Vocation	Earlier to work a. Get radio-alarm (1) b. Get time-clock for percolator (2)
	Talk with boss a. Friday noon (3)
Avocation	Regular PE program 1. Visit YMCA (5) 2. Buy copy of *Aerobics* and study (4)

Having made ultimate subdivisions, assign each a priority number, as shown above, and tackle the objectives in that order. As the goals are accomplished, mark them off. In the case of ongoing activities (study *Aerobics*), set aside a certain time of day and a certain aliquot of time and see that no lesser priorities take precedence. It is inevitable that the order of priorities change from time to time, but a good general rule is that when a conflict exists, always give precedence to the highest (or higher) priority.

Lest it seem that all life activities become reduced to a mere number in a notebook, rest assured that after the initial planning, little time is required to keep up with priorities. In a reciprocal manner to the merging of immediate goals into short-term into intermediate into long-term, long-term goals may be subdivided into intermediate into short-term and into immediate goals. For example, a bit of planning relative to the finances and security goal might result in the following tabulations (working from right to left):

Goal	**Immediate**	**Short-term**	**Intermediate**	**Long-term**
Finances and Security	Study books on: a. Land b. Stocks and bonds	Study stocks and bonds a. Investment club b. Visit brokerage house	Learn land a. Visits with realtors b. Forays into countryside c. Study country records and maps	Net Worth of $100G a. Land deals b. Stocks and bonds

Working in reverse, one can establish immediate, short-term, and intermediate goals relative to the ultimate long-term goal(s). Initally a great deal of time should be given to planning and defining long-term goals and working out tentative steps (short-term, intermediate) toward reaching those goals. Obviously the plans must be kept flexible. Detours crop up. New roads may be discovered. But at least the wheels are in orderly motion. It is the primary purpose of *priority planning* to bring order out of chaos. The modicum of time required is well worth the effort and aids immeasurably in the reduction of emotional turmoil.

Rearranging Goals

The chronically fatigued individual should take a close look at his goals from the standpoint of the qualities mentioned, with an eye to rearranging them to reduce the stress they produce or eliminating some of them if need be.

Immediacy

Failure to distinguish between immediate, short-term, intermediate, or long-term goals creates confusion and stress. Much needless jamming is the result. For example, Carol's immediate goal is to make $10,000 out of a land deal. Her long-term objective is to make a million. If she confuses the two goals and plunges too heavily into debt to try to make a killing out of her immediate goal, both goals may consequently go unrealized.

Is a goal too distant? too immediate? Has enough time been allowed to adequately tackle it? Or should it be reshuffled and placed elsewhere? Pete found that by allowing an extra year he could meet the downpayment on a new house with ease, whereas his present time schedule was causing all sorts of anxiety.

Too many immediate goals in the wrong place on a schedule may lead to a situation called *jamming*, that is so many things are occurring or are on top that a sense of utter frustration and futility prevails. Pushed to your ultimate you may simply throw up your hands and say "what's the use," with the result that nothing comes off with the precision and completeness that it should. Although such situations inevitably occur from time to time, their regular recurrence militates a reassessment of immediate goals, or else stress, anxiety, and fatigue prevail. When such situations do occur, you should meet them with a one-thing-at-a-time attitude, working steadily and assigning or reassigning priorities to the various items at hand.

Unexpected contingencies commonly contribute heavily to such situations, and there is no way you can avoid them entirely. Such days commonly arise in the life of a physician. For example, Jim's schedule on a certain day calls for: surgery, office, noon speech, office. But in midmorning a patient shows up in the emergency room with a hot appendix. Jim has to reschedule his morning patients so he can take care of the emergency before noon. The perpetual spreading of yourself too thin can yield nothing but chronic anxiety and fatigue. Careful reevaluation of your day-to-day goals is decidedly in order.

Size Rearrangement

Maybe a goal is simply too big for the time being, or it shouldn't be on the docket at all. Too large a financial goal, or too high a standard of living, for example, lead to all sorts of financial strain and stress: loans that shouldn't be obtained, mortgages that should never be signed, or extra work that taxes the capacity of the individual beyond his breaking point. One doctor's fatigue problem was eventually cured not by a physician, but by a business consultant, who found him living beyond his means and put him on a strict budget, with remarkable results.

In the setting or pursuit of a goal, you should definitely not be a hog or bite off more than you can chew. It's far better to drive a Ford in emotional comfort than a Cadillac in which one feels out of place. It's better to live in two rooms and a bath and be able to take a nice vacation now and then, than to live behind the eight ball on the top of Nob Hill.

Stepping down—reducing the size of a goal—isn't always the easiest task, in any sense of the word, especially if you have set a lot of wheels in motion: loans, commitments, intermediate goals. It's far better to be realistic about a goal in the first place. But sizing down a goal *can* be done. All it takes is facing squarely up to the situation, either through your own eyes, or through the eyes of a third party—your accountant, a business consultant or associate, your banker, your spouse—anyone who will sit down and go over your situation with you and see it like it is.

Joe was one of those chronically tired guys who worked all the overtime he could in order to meet the mortgage payments on a fine home, two autos (one for his teenaged son), and a house full of fine furnishings, as well as the initiation fee and monthly dues in a good country club in the neighborhood. His family had a ball, but Joe had only headaches, general malaise, and chronic fatigue. One day Joe took a good look at himself and went, not on a buying spree, but on a selling one. He sold his equity in everything he had—house, autos, furniture, the works—all in the face of constant furor from his not too sympathetic family. He packed up and took them with him to a remote Pacific outpost, where his only possession was a boat and motor. There, when last heard from, Joe was living like a king—fishing, scuba diving over the coral reef, and just basking on the beach. He had enough money from his sellout to last about a year, and after that Joe was going to start all over again, this time with goals that fit his pocketbook.

At first his family was furious, but in a month or two they were unwinding right along with Joe. Joe's sellout wasn't a copout at all, because in his original status Joe wasn't living; he was dying, killing himself by degrees. Sometimes radical surgery like this is necessary to cure a cancerous existence. But more often than not minor surgery will do—cutting out a goal or two, paring others down to size. Whatever the case, too many oversized goals can only wear you out.

Reassessment of Fit and Reality

Pursuing the wrong goal is like wearing an ill-fitted suit of clothes. It may look terrific in the window, but when you put it on it feels like a bag. The thing to do with goals that don't fit is to take them off and find some that do. Especially is this true of major, long-term goals, else you'll be uncomfortable for life.

How does one find goals that fit? If, by the time you are well along in a given pursuit, you haven't discovered yourself, that is recognized that you are doing what you really should be doing, you might reassess your position by taking an aptitude test designed to uncover your best potential. To find the nearest facility for such a test, contact the nearest university (psychology department), or consult a psychologist or friendly librarian.

You might also take out a correspondence course to see if your projected changeup fits your liking (it may cost you a few bucks and a few hours to find out if it does or doesn't, but that beats diving in full tilt only to find out it's another misfit). Many professions have allied fields of endeavor that offer the prospect the opportunity to get the feel of what he might be getting into. I know several women who have become licensed practical nurses well along in life because they had never had the opportunity of a career and had reached that stage when the kids were all away at school and there was that empty void so full of nothing to do. There was not time to get a nursing degree, but they got into a very useful and remunerative profession by seizing on what was available.

Friends in fields of endeavor you think you'd be interested in might introduce you, as it were, to that line of work. There's the young geologist who, disgruntled with himself after attempting to teach the subject for a year or two, visited the oil fields in tow of a friend. The outdoor life and the drama of drilling appealed to him, and now he's in the drilling business, loving every minute of it.

Still again, you might begin by making a list of some of the occupations that always interested you. Then visit a library and read up on these occupations and allied fields. It could spare you the plight of many an unhappy Dr. Kildare, his decision to study medicine illogically based on fantasy. But once you've boned up on your subject, don't stop there. Nose around in the field before you make the decision that it's for you. If law, visit courtrooms and talk with attorneys. If farming, live and work on a farm for a summer. If photography, get a job in a photographic shop. And so on. Many an occupation that looks appealing on paper, or on TV, doesn't fit when you actually give it a whirl.

Summarily, reassessing the fit of a goal revolves around an inquisitive mind. It's a lot like shopping; you spot a good-looker in the window, then try it on. You question, you probe, you search, and finally you bring to light. What with testing aids and books and communications and transportation so readily available, there is no excuse for not coming up with a good fit if you really try. What to do about changing your major goal is another subject, discussed a bit farther along.

A goal may fit and be the right one for you, but its pursuit may be unrealistic from the standpoint of life situation, finances, and such. For example, the sixty-year old carpenter who suddenly decides he'd like to be a doctor may indeed make a fine physician—the goal may fit—but the timing in life is somewhat unrealistic (although any number of older people have, indeed, studied medicine). If such a one has no other obligations and is financially able to pursue such a course, his goal is much more realistic than if he has involved family ties or must borrow the money to finance his education.

The realistic goal, if it is to be reasonably free of tension-fatigue production, fits the time, the place, the pocketbook, and circumstance. The unrealistic, artificially structured goal that does not take into account the facts of life, more often than not is a great source of stress.

Goal Definition

A well-defined goal is clear and distinct, and therefore easier to pursue and less productive of fatigue than the hazy, tenuous one. The young student who enters college in an effort to find himself—his goal(s) in life, his interests, and such—is, if he is in earnest, far more subject to emotional fatigue than the student who enters a premed course preparatory to studying medicine. In the former instance there are too many variables, nothing is clear-cut, there is no settled direction. In the latter the course is well-delineated and all the student's efforts may be concentrated upon realization of a lucid and clear-cut objective. The studious definition of a goal saves time, money, and a great deal of emotional stress in the form of frustration and fatigue.

Changing Priorities

Sometimes it turns out that in the assignment of priorities, you have put the cart before the horse. And when such becomes evident, you need to change priorities. For example, Stuart's top priority for an intermediate goal was assigned to moving into a new house two years after he got out on his own. His second priority was to get a promotion within that same period. After a few months it became evident that in order to carry out priority 1, priority 2 was going to have to come to pass first. Accordingly, he changed priorities, applied some of his house savings to a program of night study at a nearby college, and got his promotion. After that, the new house came easy.

Another frequent reason to change priorities is the exigency, the unexpected, the "bridge out" or "detour" sign that suddenly confronts us when we turn the corner. Like Stuart, Rose and Mack had their eyes on a new house in a year or two—priority 1—and after that a family cruiser—priority 2. Instead they found out they were having a baby. As it turned out they had to change their priority from boats to babies. They could have tried to hang on to all three, but the resultant stress on their salaries wouldn't have been worth it. So they simply moved the boat from a short to a long-term goal, and had plenty of time and money to enjoy their child.

When time schedules don't come off, due to exigencies, circumstance, or whatever, don't hesitate to shuffle goals to new priorities of immediacy. Moving the new house back a couple of years, or three, or five; buying that farm four or five years later than anticipated; investing in a new office building in four years instead of two; beats tying yourself up in knots just for the sake of staying on schedule. Trying to do too many things too soon is almost certain to produce an aura of chronic stress with its handmaidens of anxiety and fatigue. Rather than pushing your purse and buying that new Fireball Eight, take heed of the recession, get that motor overhauled on your old Saturn Six, and settle down in it for a couple of more years of ulcerless driving.

Don't be afraid to reshuffle the deck. And don't let pride or stubbornness overrule reason. Your neighbor may look down his nose at you when you drive by in that four-year-old car, but you can laugh when he is driving by in his new one on the way to the doctor.

Changing Direction

There are usually several routes to the top of a mountain, and the same is true for most goals. If the route you chose originally proves too long or too circuitous, move to another one if the effort required doesn't outweigh the benefits of the move. Or, on the other hand, if the path you're on is too steep (even though it may be shorter), move over to a less precipitous (though longer) one. The object is to get to the top, and the route you choose is incidental.

A couple of doctors, tops in their specialty, found themselves woefully short of funds at the end of their first two years in medical school. Borrowing money to foot the bills would have proved a tremendous strain. So they got part-time jobs at the school and spread their last two years work over four years. They may have been dubbed "chronics" by some of the guys, but they got their M.D. degree and had a relaxed time doing it. Flexibility of thinking is essential in this phase of goal manipulation.

Reassessing Current Values

With the passage of time, or the advent of the unexpected, goals set years ago (or months) become outdated and even worthless. On the other hand, some become more valuable. In other words, goal values change. Hence the need to constantly reevaluate goals in the light of what has transpired and is transpiring in a life pattern.

Evelyn's immediate goal of moving into a house rather than an apartment became meaningless when her husband suddenly became ill and required a major operation. Membership in a certain country club was removed from an M.D.'s list when her company told her she might be transferred to another city. Dave's goal of a retirement fund of $100,000 seemed ample ten years ago, but with inflation rampant that figure had to be doubled.

On the other side of the coin, the completion of a home machine shop by Bob seemed at first a third-rate priority. But in the course of a few years a healthy sideline business had developed, such that Bob could foresee changing his avocation to his vocation. Hence it became necessary to give first priority to what was once an afterthought.

As goal values change, so does priority. Only an ostrich attitude fails to take changing values into due consideration, with resultant stress and strain that could easily have been avoided.

CHAPTER 15

Altering the Physical Environment

In the previous chapter you considered alterations of goal(s) as a means of reducing stress, and therefore tension-fatigue. Here you shall consider alteration of the environment to achieve the same end. Again, although overlap exists, let us consider such alterations from physical, mental, and emotional aspects.

The first question that you must ask in this regard is: what can I do with my physical surroundings to make them more enjoyable, increase my efficiency, aid rest (reduce stress and therefore tension-fatigue), and decrease depressive factors. You might ask of your home for example: could I redo a room or two in more cheerful decor? What about a bright painting on the wall? Could the air-conditioning be improved upon? Would a humidifier be of value? Or how about a new mattress? even a new bed? Or how about just moving to a new locale with more pleasant surroundings?

Karen and Roy lived near a busy airport, which grew not only busier but noisier. Eventually the noise factor became so great that sleep was hard to come by, and their jobs and home life began to suffer. So they sold their house—at a loss—but what they lost monetarily they gained in tranquility and made back in efficiency.

Or how about, in extreme cases, just changing environments entirely, like the asthma patient who moves from a damp, humid section of the country to a hot, dry one?

At work many of the same considerations apply. Is the lighting adequate? the ventilation? Is the noise factor too great? Are irritant fumes too bothersome? For most problems there are solutions. But first the problem must be recognized and identified.

Obstacles in the environment between you and your goal must be removed or altered for the better if they are a source of stress. Such obstacles may be either tangible or intangible. An example of the former was Dorothy's automobile, a vintage model, thoroughly undependable, requiring costly maintenance bills, and costing Dorothy any number of dockings for tardiness, not to mention her being in a constant stew from wrestling with the device. A little arithmetic showed Dorothy that it was false economy to nurse this tin can along, so she spruced it up, sold it for a pretty penny, and acquired a dependable iron horse in its place.

Mike provides an example of the latter, in this case a distance factor. He lived across town from his work. At best it required an hour's tussle with traffic to make it to work each A.M. and back again in the evening. The result was a work record moth-eaten with tardiness and no-shows. The solution was simple: shorten the distance to and from work, which he could do either by moving closer to his present job or getting a job closer to home. Since he had been with his company many years, he chose the former route, and found himself far less fatigued at the end of the day.

CHAPTER 16

Altering the Mental Environment

Alteration of the mental environment to reduce chronic stress involves rendering our surroundings more conducive to learning, thought, and appreciation or enjoyment of the more pleasant sensory stimuli available to us.

The habitual use of extant library facilities in the community, attendance at schools or seminars, the ready use of correspondence courses, study clubs, regular reading habits, pay TV, or the acquisition of a good home library are all means available to most persons bent on improving the mental framework of their lives. That half-used storage space in the attic may, with a bit of ingenuity, be converted into a most useful and beneficial library, study, or workroom.

Blank wall space may be converted into reminders, via plaques and posters and prints, of the reward of mental effort. A tape recorder is an excellent means of carrying lecture material into the bathroom, the garage, down the highway—wherever—and converting wasted time into highly constructive minutes. Taking along meaningful reading material in your briefcase, when periods of waiting can be anticipated, is an excellent means of improving the mind.

Many persons under chronic stress, and therefore subject to chronic fatigue, seem totally unaware of areas in life other than the one in which they live and move and have their being. The scientist lives with his nose in a test tube, the engineer with a computer in his pocket, the accountant with a pencil behind his ear, and so on. That there are other areas in which the mind may indulge itself for surcease from the day-to-day turmoil never seems to occur to them. They suffer, as it were, from telescopic vision, seeing only what they have been trained to see, or to hear, and no more. Such persons must learn to broaden their horizons. The ear that is accustomed to hear only sales and service must be retrained to hear great music. The eye that sees only what the microscope sees must be educated to see and appreciate the handiwork of great artists. The mind that stores only facts and figures must learn to wander through the pages of great literature.

With radio, TV (certain programs), and library availability what it is today, there is no excuse for anyone's not availing himself of such training. Art museums are quite ubiquitous. Hi-fi equipment is within the reach of practically every pocketbook. A tape deck for the automobile might prove a much more profitable investment than an automobile telephone. Book clubs are very reasonable. And so on. The way out of the mental doldrums is limited only by the imagination of the individual.

CHAPTER 17

Altering the Emotional Environment

Most emotional stress in adults emanates from or is related to (1) the job, (2) the home, or (3) the peer group. Thus alterations in one or all of these spheres are essential to reduction of emotional stress.

The Job

Feelings about work give rise to all sorts of emotions, some good, some bad. Thomas Carlyle labeled "blessed. . .he who has found his work," and James Lowell "blessed. . .the horny hands of toil." It was Thomas Dekker who gave to "honest labor. . .a lovely face," and Robert Louis Stevenson who concluded that "true success is. . .to labor." But Charles Lamb decried "who first invented work. . .and tied the free. . .rejoicing spirit down to the ever-haunting importunity of business. . ." The divine fiat that man work six days out of seven undoubtedly foresaw that work is the very staff of life, the stuff of which living is fashioned. But not all men or women accept the decree gracefully, and the varied emotions which are generated by a job situation in any given individual lend credence to the statement that "no job remains the same when it changes hands." Thus gut feelings about jobs are probably as individual as fingerprints.

The complexities of job situations in modern industrialized societies, geared as they are to the clock and the calendar and the masses, make for infinitely more problem areas than the situations which existed in an agrarian economy. Speed, efficiency, and pressure-packed schedules have become the order of the day as the plow has given way to the pen, and the trowel to the telephone. And with complexity job tensions have increased, until nowadays work-associated tension has been found to affect some five of every six male laborers in the U.S. Admittedly job-related tensions are to some extent inevitable, yet if improperly managed or out of proportion they may become disabling. Satisfaction with your occupation is inextricably linked to good health and longevity, a most important observation when it is further recognized that, although most people learn to cope with stress on the job, relatively few, given the opportunity for an out, would continue to work out of sheer enjoyment of their job.

As pointed out in an excellent article, "Coping with Occupational and Organizational Stress,"* a number of elements, such as fit of the job, over-

*R.L. Kahn, G.V. Coelho, and D.A. Hamburg, "Coping with Occupational and Organizational Stress," *Medical Tribune* (28 May 1975) pp. 13-20, (Nutley, N.J.: Roche Laboratories, Division of Hoffman-LaRoche Inc.) By permission.

load, role conflict, ambiguity, and boredom ultimately determine the degree of satisfaction or dissatisfaction with a job, and must be dealt with accordingly. Reduced to ultimate simplicity the ideal job situation (seldom encountered in real life) consists of the right job for the right person at the right time. Let's look at these items a little more closely.

The Right Job

Certain job properties, such as flexibility (opportunity for advancement or change), good environment, and the proper load of demands and responsibilities are essential to ultimate satisfaction with any job.

Job Flexibility

Being in a job rut with no chance of getting out is akin to being in a straitjacket. It's a stressful experience that breeds a great deal of inner tension. A good job offers the opportunity to move either forward or sideways—which is to say that if you cannot move up in the organization, you can at least find a diversity of activities, preferably of a challenging nature. The person who feels helplessly boxed in to a stereotyped routine may have to obtain relief by seeking out some new challenge or variation of his job situation. For example, Sandy experienced a great deal of fatigue when engaged in the routine posting of charges in a bookkeeping office. But when allowed the person-to-person contact of working with collections, his job took on a new flavor, and his fatigue greatly improved.

Job Environment

The environment of a job may have a great deal to do with imposed stress. I have alluded elsewhere to physical environment, but to cite yet another example, a person subject to asthma whose illness is aggravated by working in a paint factory would obviously do well to get out of the paint factory.

The mental environment of a job may likewise be a source of dissatisfaction and stress. Ellen liked animals and, while awaiting entry to veterinary school, got a job in the boarding kennels at a medical school. But she also had a highly inquisitive mind and, after a few weeks, her job took on an aura of drudgery. When she asked for and received permission to assist in animal surgery, the drudgery and the tired-of-the-routine element took wings.

Finally the emotional environment of a job situation may play the most important role of all; such environment is the product of interaction of your personality with those of your coworkers', a formula which makes for all sorts of pressure problems. Consider for example, the "sandwich syndrome," a dilemma from which almost half of all American workers suffer.*Here the worker finds himself attempting to satisfy the demands of two or more superiors, a situation which necessitates that the worker confront

*Ibid.

those who have put him in the middle with the impossibility of his situation, or if need be, go over some heads and secure an arbiter. Still another twixt-a-rock-and-a-hard-place situation may arise when a person must satisfy the customers of his company while at the same time fulfilling contrary expectations of his own management. An individual who finds himself in such a position at frequent intervals must frequently choose between a job change and an ulcer, tension headaches, or high blood pressure—and the attendant fatigue—unless, that is, he becomes expert enough to anticipate conflicts and think out solutions ahead of time. Sharing problems of this type with other employees in similar situations often helps a great deal. Ed, a very good salesman for a hardware firm, often found himself in just such a quandary. He worked for a very demanding company and had to put in long hours catering to equally demanding clients. Fatigue and an ulcer became Ed's ever-present companions. Confrontation with management yielded only an impasse. And he could not buck his clientele and maintain his good sales record. His solution? He changed jobs.

Demands and Responsibilities

The job load should be of the right magnitude both as it relates to the *amount* of work to be done within a given time (quantitative load*) and the *kind* of work to be done (qualitative load*) by a given individual. As tax-return deadlines approach, tax accountants frequently find themselves faced with "more than they can say grace over." They may know their job well, but there simply may be too much to do, whereupon the midnight oil burns long and late, tension mounts, and the diseases of maladaptation (ulcers, high blood pressure, asthma, etc.) surface and thrive. Fatigue is the almost constant handmaiden of such endeavor. Too much of the wrong kind of a job might be typified by the high school math teacher asked to substitute in a biology class for which he was ill-prepared because of inadequate training. Though he did the job (via pre-class cramming), he suffered a series of vascular headaches as a result. A job which demands too much simply because there is not enough time (that is there is no shortage of physical and mental capabilities) should be divided up or passed around. In short get more hands or heads. If this is not possible, then you should organize your time well with regards to priorities and assume a dogged one-thing-at-a-time attitude. If the job is too much because of inadequate training, experience, or ability (comparable to a nonswimmer's falling into water over his head), then the swimmer should call for help (yield to someone who can do the job) or learn to swim (that is where time and opportunity permit, upgrade your ability to do the job).

Lucidity

The right job also possesses the quality of *lucidity,* that is what is expected of you is crystal clear, with no gray areas. Imprecise, poorly defined

*Ibid.

duties leave you befuddled and uncertain, and hence tense and tired. You may want to perform brilliantly and may well be able to do so, but lacking clear-cut guidelines, you may act hesitantly or not at all. As pointed out by Dr. Kahn,* murky, ambiguous tasks, even though associated with little personal risk, are much more prone to produce stress than potentially dangerous jobs in which procedures are clearly defined. A good example of this, says Dr. Kahn, is the astronaut. He may experience relatively little stress in the flight of his hazardous but well-delineated mission when compared to the ground crew supervisor, whose many ill-defined contingencies, for which he is ultimately responsible, stress him severely. Many a job could be converted from a tension-filled fatiguing one to a pleasant, relaxing one by the simple expedient of the employer spelling out to you precisely what your job duties are. If necessary, written manuals of procedure should be compiled. One refinery lab foreman that I knew was able to increase the efficiency of his lab crew considerably by just such a procedure, and much to his surprise, his workers expressed considerably more job satisfaction after they had written down their job responsibilities and gone over them with the foreman.

The Right Person

The right person for a given job is one with the proper combination of genes and training to fill that particular slot. Human beings arrive on planet earth with genetic equipment from which various personality types emerge. At one end of the spectrum is the nervous Nellie type—high-strung, time-conscious, and habitually straining at the leash. At the other end is phlegmatic Freddie—always calm and composed, never in a hurry, loose as a wet noodle. In between these extremes lie all sorts of admixtures and gradations of the two.

Doctors Rosenman and Friedman** have labeled the tense, time-conscious, overly ambitious, driver-type personality as Type A, and found such persons subject to a high rate of heart attacks. The easy-going individual, who tends to shun clocks and calendars, has been called a Type B and found far less likely to suffer a coronary episode. If the tension-fatigue associated with a job is to be minimized, nervous Nellies (Type As) would do better to shy away from demanding schedules and time-oriented jobs, while the phlegmatic Freddies, as a group, would actually turn in a better performance, from a fatigue standpoint, in more stimulating situations. This is particularly true if the training of a given individual ill prepares him for the job situation into which he may be thrust. Contrariwise, good preparation can, to some extent, overcome the genetic pattern, such that highly trained

*Ibid.

**M. Friedman and R.H. Rosenman, *Type A Behavior and Your Heart* (New York: Knopf, 1974).

nervous Nellies might never be satisfied to do anything less than what they have been expertly trained to do, even though the job may be of Type A category.

Sally's first job was as an apprentice in a clinical laboratory. She was a perfectionist, high-strung, and full of energy, but she experienced "jamming," a sort of frenetic inertia of rest, when the work piled up. She grew anxious and always tired and, thinking that married life was the life for her, accepted the first offer of marriage. But married life, filled with comparatively little to do, soon grew dull and routine, not for her set of genes. So she returned to the laboratory, but this time by way of an excellent training course which enabled her to deal much more effectively with the work at hand. She was sailing along in a happy state when last heard of. This is an example of what proper training can do to alter the gene effect in a given individual.

In the final analysis, you must be fitted to the job as much as the job to you. To neglect consideration of personality types and genetic equipment is to overlook at least half of the formula for job satisfaction.

The Right Time

A given job may be just right for you at one time in your life, and all wrong at another. To wit, Linda was a doctor who, early in her practice, developed a strong dislike for the telephone and confining schedules. So strong, in fact, that she left private practice to become an insurance physician. Though not so remunerative, the insurance business suited her to a T, in that nights and weekends were her own, and her schedule lax enough that she could read and fish more or less at will. But after many years, the insurance routine became dull and fatiguing and monotonous, enough so that Linda (in her late fifties when she did so) left the insurance business to train in psychiatry, and is once again finding her work rewarding.

Again single bliss may allow you to enjoy a job that the demands of marriage (on time, money, and what not) would not, so that a perfectly enjoyable job before marriage may be converted into a stressful one afterwards (though just the opposite may be true, of course).

A young person in the vigor of youth may be able to handle a demanding job with ease, a job which would, if tackled later in life, be the cause of inestimable stress. On the flip side of this coin, however, is the adeptness and smoothness which long years of experience bring to an occupation, with an attendant minimum of new-job stress and fatigue which are so common to greenhorns.

Incomplete training for a given task may be just as stressful as no training at all, and the person who pulls up short of completing his training in order to get into the money in a hurry commonly pays the price of tension and fatigue. Another doctor, for example, plunged into a specialty practice before he had completed his residency, though he had full intention of going back and finishing some day. The dollars began to roll in, and for a number of years Milt felt he had made a good decision. But with time he found himself up against highly trained specialists in his field, as well as being denied membership on hospital staffs and in organizations open only to fully accredited physicians. Tension and fatigue began to dog him, and not until he completed his training (at a rather late age in life) did he feel at ease again. The moral is that when humanly possible (and it usually *is* possible), your training should be full and complete before you embark on a highly specialized occupation or profession. The extra effort pays handsome dividends in satisfaction and freedom from anxiety.

Miscellaneous Job Considerations

Getting a Promotion

A promotion can be a real ego trip for the person who has stalled out, that is gone as far as he can in his particular job. He suddenly finds new energy for new tasks in place of the tiring, repetitive job he has learned to do with his eyes closed. Jack was brilliant when it came to machinery, and it didn't take long for him to feel harnessed when confined to an assembly line in a food-processing plant. It was only after promotion to the maintenance department, where he could make use of his natural talent for coping with obstreperous machines, that he fell in love with his job and lost the strange fatigue that gripped him on the assembly line.

Misplacement

As stated, a satisfying job, like a well-tailored suit of clothes, fits the individual—his personality, capabilities and capacities, and training and background. While few people are actually in love with their jobs, most persons find them sufficiently intriguing to continue at them without disabling fatigue. Occasionally, however, truly square pegs show up in round holes; such a worker, a total misfit for his job, may, due to lack of motivation, eventually find it almost impossible to get out of bed each morning. Consider Sheila, trained to the nth degree in engineering. Unable to find a job in her chosen field, she took a job as a shoe saleswoman. Complete inability to adjust to such a task forced Sheila to solve her problem by returning to school and getting a teaching certificate, whereupon she taught math and science until an engineering position opened up.

Boredom

I have already dealt with monotony in Chapter 11. Suffice it to say that monotony and lack of imagination are the name of the game with a high percentage of jobs. Most persons endure such jobs, simply assuming a neutral attitude toward them. Such boredom, as you have seen, may be attacked in a variety of ways: using the job as a means to an end; accepting it for its pay and security; concentrating on aspects of the job other than the work itself (for example, on the workers at hand); social interactions; concentrating on diversions (break times, lunch time organized athletic activities among the workers); and injecting meaning or creativity into the job.

Job Loss

A Johns Hopkins professor has shown a direct link between unemployment and stress-related illnesses. Death from stroke and heart and kidney disease rise with the loss of jobs. The person who has lost his job is faced with an extremely stressful experience. His ego is crushed. It is imperative that such a person remain physically active, utilizing such outlets as sports when no other outlet is available. The mind likewise must be kept occupied, not with anxiety, but with worthwhile pursuits. An automobile engineer, during a layoff, began using his knowledge of auto mechanics to repair ailing neighborhood autos in his garage and had soon developed a thriving referral business. A laid-off factory worker parlayed his love for fishing into a full-time fishing-guide business; he still guides for fun and profit when his regular job allows. It is not at all an uncommon experience for a person to come out of a layoff in a better situation than he was in, provided he keeps his head on straight and puts the mind to work.

Of utmost importance is that if you are jobless you face up to your problem, realize that there are alternatives, and actively seek and find them. Alterations in the job picture of either a minor or major nature may be necessary. The most important attributes of the jobless worker should be a flexibility and willingness to make a change.

Minor Alterations

Minor alterations consist of altering the work picture within the organization, by improving or changing skills, by altering relationships with superiors, by injecting diversionary activity, and so on. It is of foremost importance that you identify and clarify your source(s) of stress, assess the avenues of correction or alteration open to you, and act accordingly.

Major Alterations

Major alterations are found in promotions, sometimes demotions, a relocation within the organization, or sometimes, quitting and starting all over again. As regards the latter move, there may be more to be said for it, in terms of tension relief, than most other measures. It is admittedly drastic, however, and should be resorted to only when all else fails to yield relief, and when such a move is logical and carefully thought out. Remember Sam, the human dynamo? Many a Sam is such a victim of routine and accumulated mortgage debts that he is on a virtual treadmill, and must (so he thinks), wend his weary way around in order to survive. But every once in a while one reads of a Sam who wakes up to his plight.

Doctor Harvey, for example, was burdened down by the ever-mounting and continual pressures of private practice in a big city. He had accumulated mountainous mortgages and was a slave to a high and expensive echelon of social-cultural activity. And he was forever tired. When he wound up in the hospital with a bleeding ulcer, he had time to think. Was he really living? or was he merely holding down a seat in a pressure tank? His kids were out of school and his decision was easy. On leaving the hospital, he put everything he owned up for sale, including his practice. Three months later he was an insurance doctor in a resort city, where he worked eight-hour days, no nights, no weekends, and had more time off than he knew what to do with (at first). The pay was considerably less, but Doctor Harvey got to know his wife for the first time. His fatigue disappeared and he felt ten years younger. He became an expert fisherman and never ceased to be amazed when he looked back upon the tiresome web he had spun for himself in his first life.

Doctor Bob was in a similar situation, only his out was entirely away from medicine. He became a horse wrangler on a dude ranch and fell in love with the out-of-doors and the freedom from pressure. There isn't enough money in the world, he says, to lure him back to his pressure cooker.

What most Sams don't realize, or won't realize, is that there *are* alternatives to slavery to a pressure-packed way of life. You only have to look for them. You must first properly assess your situation and then act accordingly. Frequently there are choices involved—more money or more time? a big house or one that is merely adequate? the social whirlpool or the trout pool in the nearby stream? In the final analysis, Sam must change his philosophy of life. In the words of Thoreau:

> If a man does not keep pace with his companions,
> Perhaps it is because he hears a different drummer.
> Let him step to the music which he hears,
> However measured or far away.

The Home

In cases of chronic fatigue, the home environment should be conducive to rest and freedom from stress. "A man's home is his castle" applies here as perhaps in no other sphere. Ideally the home is surrounded by a "moat of tranquility" which enables us to retreat regularly from the pressures and the mad scramble of the workaday world. Unfortunately such is all too often not the case, and when we cross the moat to the castle, we merely exchange one type of stress for another. The cauldron of unrest that boils so flagrantly in so many homes nowadays is fueled, basically, from four different reservoirs: (1) interpersonal relationships, (2) boundary relationships, (3) family goals, and (4) role fulfillment.

Interpersonal Relationships

The relationships between husband and wife, wife and children, and father and children determine, to a major extent, the general atmosphere of the home. Hostilities, suspicions, distrust, disrespect, and lack of consideration between family members can only lead to tension. Mutual love, respect, and consideration one for the other are basic to a peaceful milieu. Without these latter ingredients, family harmony and, therefore, unity, are impossible to achieve. A recognition of the importance of relationships is essential to an overall grasp of the chronic fatigue problem.

Boundary Relationships

Inadvertently what happens to various family members outside the home affects attitudes and dispositions within the home. The parent whose job is insecure commonly lends an air of insecurity to the family circle. The parent who has been snubbed socially not uncommonly snubs loved ones in return. The child who is in jeopardy of failing his school work may likewise fail to live up to his responsibilities at home. And what affects one family member in this regard always affects other family members. It is impossible to isolate a problem inside the "castle." Contagion is inevitable and certain, and attempts to secrete difficulties from one another serve only to compound the created stress. Truly, within the home, "no man is an island unto himself."

Family Goals

Family goals determine to a large extent the direction and purpose of various family activities. For example, the health-oriented family may jog or cycle together. The family with a financial goal may find it necessary for one or more parent to work at an extra job. The family seeking a certain social status may find themselves pushed to keep the children in a special school. And so on. Family goals are desirable, but as with individual goals, must frequently be reassessed by the family if they are unrealistic or too demanding, creating excessive stress and strife.

Role Fulfillment

The woman in the family wants to be a good mother and a good wife. The man desires to be a good father and a good husband. And the child, it is to be hoped, desires to be a good child. So long as the individual feels that he is fulfilling the home role assigned, he experiences a deep inner satisfaction which overflows into his relationships with the various family members. When such a role is, for one or another reason, thwarted, frustrated, or otherwise brought up short, the inner dissatisfaction and tension resulting in that individual makes itself felt all up or down the line. Success within the family unit is dependent upon the success of *all* family members carrying out their expected duties. Failure here is as contagious as the measles within those same walls.

Basic Determinants of Home Stress

The foundational determinants of stress (or conversely of tranquility) within the home are background (hereditary and environmental) and training of the occupants. The attitudes, beliefs, and motivational factors which determine the conduct of a given individual in a given situation are a composite of what that person was born with genetically and what he was taught in his formative years (home, church, and school), and what he received in the way of formal training in later years (peers, college, professional schools, special schools, self-help).

Computer-determined marriages have been found to have a high degree of success, a fact which, if true, can be related to the rational elimination of divergent factors in two individuals and the matchup of convergent ones. Such a matchup, at least mathematically, has a far greater probability of success than a chance mating. For the probability that any two persons of different backgrounds and training, both in quantity as well as quality, will see eye to eye on all important aspects of life is indeed infinitesimal when left to chance. But even the computer cannot erase all divergences of opinion.

Alterations in Home Pressures

Alterations in the home scene must be away from friction and toward harmony between all members of the family unit. If the family unit has a toothache (for example, a child is unhappy in school), it should no more be ignored than if it has a heart attack (parent loses a job). As a unit, the family may need to adjust its status level, which may mean giving up some things for the sake of lessening tension. It may need to refine its goals, reassign priorities, and reevaluate its true worth. Such assessments must often begin with the individual, who must learn that his wishes must be subservient to the welfare of the family as a whole. Frequently this requires self-aid, group therapy, or even professional help.

The recognition that the home environment may be one of constant tension or of ready relaxation is essential to the chronically tired individual. And again such recognition must be followed up by whatever action is necessary to relieve tension in this critical area. The father, the mother, and the child in today's pressure-packed society must have a stable, serene home base from which to operate. Without it there can be no more hope for successful coping with the tensions of life than for a general's fighting a successful battle on two fronts. The home must be a retreat for rest and recreation from the inevitable and inexorable battles raging without.

Peer Pressure

Peer pressure, in today's society, is an exceedingly important source of environmental stress. The pressure to achieve, to win, to advance, and to acquire may emanate from organizations (job, club, lodges, schools), social groups, or even recreational activities. Were it not for peer pressure, the Sams of our society would be far fewer in number, for it is the peer who provides the basis for comparison, who flings the gauntlet, who all too often sets the goal. In primitive, close-knit societies (where the emphasis is on group security) stress illnesses, such as ulcers, hypertension, and colitis, are practically unheard of. In such societies internal competition is absent. It is the group against the environment without, rather than the individual against environment without and within. In such societies what one person achieves, all achieve; what is sought for the good of one, is sought for the good of all. Goals are unified and distinct and simple, rather than individualized and complex and often hazy. The pressures are group pressures, and they are distributed evenly amongst all members of the group. One member does not forge ahead socially, for example, and thus set a goal for another member of his group. All move ahead together. All strive equally for common goals. Contrast this with a highly industrialized society, in which a man's success is measured by how he measures up to the accomplishments, the bank account, the status of his neighbor, his coworker, or his weekend buddy. The Sams of our day are all too often but small cogs in a big wheel, and they go round and round simply because the wheel turns.

Achievement

The American people are, as a whole, hooked on achievement. Achievement is a hallmark of success, and recognition the badge for admission into the top echelon of our society. The young child learns from family, friends, and teachers that if he is to be anything at all, he must start climbing the ladder at an early age and never stop climbing. Job satisfaction is uncommon, not only because of square pegs in round holes, but because there are higher levels to reach. Sam will never be satisfied with an Econo-Six, simply because the Fireball-Eight is the best. He has friends who own one, and the TV commercials and the magazine ads subtly suggest that he has not arrived until he owns one. So the heat is on to advance along all fronts—financial, social, job, whatever. Onward and upward is the battle cry that spurs the Sams of our day to plunge madly into their concrete-and-steel jungles day after day, month after month, year after year. For in achieving is advancement, and with advancement comes acquisition, and with acquisition wealth and power.

Joe was a loan officer in a bank. He often golfed with Jim, a vp in the same institution, at Jim's club. Joe always came away feeling just a little bit inferior and a little bit snubbed, even though Jim never mentioned his higher position in the bank. The net result was that Joe always felt tense around Jim, and by comparison, unhappy with his position.

Mary was a member of a bridge club where she often played at a table with Susie. Susie, a highschool friend, had made a successful career in television producing. Mary had an unexciting job in a bank. Susie wore new fashions and gold jewelry, while Mary sported old clothes and costume jewelry. Mary felt uncomfortable, tense, and tired after her bridge sessions, and because to her husband she openly compared her status to that of Susie's, she made her husband tense as well.

The pursuit of life, liberty, and happiness becomes, early in life, the pursuit of the dollar and the scepter. No man is content to merely "catch up with the Joneses." He must pass them. And the pressures entailed—the eternal hustle and bustle, the clanging and the haranguing, the push and the pull—be hanged. Sam is going to make it or bust, and his tensions and his fatigue will just have to wait.

Winning

The six-year old was sporting a T-shirt which read: Losing is a No-No. His older sister, on the tennis court beside which the boy stood, was playing a high school tournament match as if her life depended on it. When in agony she netted the last point in defeat, she emitted a shrill moan and flung her racket over the fence behind her. Like thousands and thousands of other youngsters across this great nation of ours, the girl had been taught, from toddler age on up, that the name of the game in this life is winning, at all costs.

A famous coach of recent years said, "Winning is not a sometime thing. You don't win once in a while, you don't do things right once in a while, you do them right all the time. Winning is a habit. Unfortunately so is losing. There is no room for second place. There is only one place in my game and that is first."

Harvard sociologist Seymour Lipset recently stated that, "In the United States, the thing that matters is who wins, no matter how. There is more emphasis on accomplishing something, no matter what means are used."

While there is nothing inherently wrong with the desire to win, the desire to do your best at whatever you undertake, there is everything wrong with making no allowance for losing, whether at an athletic contest, a business deal, or a national election. What is important in our society is not how you played the game, but did you win? The toddler, the preschool child, the Little Leaguer, the high school contestant, and eventually the business and professional man find themselves prodded and goaded, ruthlessly and inexorably, by family, teacher, and finally their peers to be a winner. What anxieties, what tensions, what frustrations develop and mount in the Sams of this nation who have not the necessary tools, hereditary or otherwise, to be a winner! Failing to see the virtue in simply doing their best, the satisfaction to be derived from doing well whatever task they can perform, the reward of constant effort, they are marked by their peers, and often by themselves, as losers. And the resultant load of anxiety, tension, and fatigue grows ever greater, eventually robbing our Sams of whatever chance they may have had of an enjoyable life.

What a pity that the little Sams in our midst cannot be taught to compete for the joy of competing and cannot be spared the ignominy of losing. Instead we would make Babe Ruths of all our Little League baseballers, Red Granges of all of our little halfbacks, and Chris Everts of our little racqueteers. What a shame that financial success is measured by the standard of an Andrew Mellon or an Aristotle Onassis rather than a comfortable income at a comfortable pace. What a shame that job success is measured by how many placques of recognition a man has received, how many promotions are his, at what new levels he is shooting, rather than by the satisfaction of doing whatever job he does well. Although such peer attitudes may emanate from the heritage of being an American, a citizen of a country born of strife, where winning or losing meant life or death as a nation, this does not alter the fact that the vast majority of our citizenry are also-rans—losers, if you will—in the eyes of their peers. And the handmaiden of being an also-ran is stress, anxiety, and fatigue.

Coping with Peer Pressure

Basically there are only two mechanisms for dealing with peer pressure. One is by changing peers, the other by changing one's outlook or philosophy. The person who feels uncomfortable, stressed, and anxious as a result of peer relationships should not hesitate to change peer groups if that is what it takes to relieve the stress.

Daniel was a salesman for a high-powered furniture manufacturer. Comparisons of PQs (performance quotients) were constantly made between various salesmen in the organization, such that in order to feel secure and put up a good front, Daniel spent long hours on the road, away from home and family. He found himself more intent on coming up with a good PQ than in enjoying his job, which, originally, he had liked a great deal. Pressures became so great that Daniel quit the fireball outfit and joined an older, more established company in which individual comparisons were not so flagrant. His tensions and fatigue immediately lessened, and life took on some meaning beside maintaining a high PQ.

Barbara was a member of an elite country club, most of whose members had net worths in the seven-figure range. She found herself constantly pressured to go in on deals which were out of her financial range, and when she did not do so, she could almost feel the disdain of club friends. Eventually she quit the Uptown Club and joined the Downtowner instead. There she met members who could talk her language at her level and with whom she could participate and express herself freely. For the first time in her life, Barbara's club life became a source of relaxation rather than tension.

Changing peer groups may seem to some to be the chicken way out. Not so. Often it is the smart way out. For, in reality, no one makes a peer his judge except that individual himself. And in stress situations you should no more mind changing peer groups than changing a suit of clothes. If you find cold climates to your dislike, you should move to warmer climes. If you find that chocolate gives you the hives, then you should switch to a different dessert. If red is not your color, then change to blue. And so on. It's that simple. The individual who voluntarily remains in a stressful peer relationship, when alternatives exist, is comparable to a man willfully hitting himself on the head with a hammer instead of switching to a comfortable massage.

But what can you do if you find it necessary to remain in a stressful peer situation? There is only one thing to do: change your philosophy and roll with the punches. You must recognize that if doing your level best is not good enough for your peers, then it *is* good enough for you. Being snubbed is, though sometimes humiliating, nevertheless painless and inconsequential; your own inward serenity is ultimately not determined by the opinions of the Johns and Jills that surround you, but by your opinion of yourself. "To thine own self be true, and the devil-take-the-hindmost" becomes your motto, of necessity. That your peer group may make or break you becomes of secondary concern. Your attention is focused on doing your best under whatever circumstances.

Rational man can ask no more of anyone than that. And you can most assuredly ask no more of yourself. The person in a forced peer situation does his duty as he sees it and, beyond that, holds no fear of what irrational man can do to him. In short, he derives his satisfaction from within rather than without. Here a great deal of one's personal philosophy of life is involved, and I shall have more to say of this in the next chapter.

CHAPTER 18

Altering Your Response

With regard to the reduction of stress in a life situation, you have thus far looked at the goal and the environment. Let us now consider what steps may be taken to better equip you to deal with stress.

Get Rid of Excess Baggage

Just as obesity represents excess physical baggage, so do mental and emotional hangups represent excess emotional baggage. Undue emphasis of minor emotional problems, for example, can carry over into problems of major concern and interfere with maximum mental efficiency, thus compounding tension and fatigue. For example, Gail's little tiffs with her husband were of such concern to her that she frequently found herself unable to concentrate on her office work and, in conferences, found herself thinking of her domestic problems rather than paying attention to business. The result was decreased efficiency at her job, which in turn led to job problems that added to tension-fatigue. Gail needs to recognize that minor disagreements in the home are not unusual, that they are best dealt with at home, and that, just as one should not carry business home, one should also not carry home problems to work. In short, Gail's marital difficulties, of minor proportions as they were, were simply excess baggage for her to carry to work.

Sometimes neurotic tendencies tend to crop up in similar fashion. To illustrate, Mary, on returning home from work one day, found that she had left the oven on in her kitchen; the heat was terrific and the finish on the stove had been ruined, though no serious damage had been done. Thereafter she found herself sitting and wondering, while at work, if she had remembered to turn off the oven, although she knew quite well that she had. Mary was suffering from a compulsion which, if unable to be dispelled by her own efforts, might well require professional help.

Such hangups are analogous to an elephant hunter so busy taking pot shots at rats and mice that he fails to see the elephant go by; or the baseball pitcher so intent on the man at first that he lets the runner at third base steal home. If stress, and therefore tension-fatigue, is to be properly dealt with, such emotional thorns must go, either by way of self-discipline or by way of whatever help from the outside may be necessary.

In a similar vein you must discipline yourself to giving full attention to whatever bona fide problem is at hand. For example, if she neglects it, Gail's marital problem, of minor proportions now, might blossom into one of major degree. And if she fails to leave her domestic problems out of her business problems, the result may well be disaster in two areas instead of one. If the surgeon's mind is on a business deal while performing an operation, he can do neither job to the best of his ability. Such cases of "divided attention" are characteristic of poor mental discipline, and it is no wonder that the practitioners of such dual mentality are often tense and fatigued. "One thing at a time," and "each at the proper time" *must* become the watchword of the victim of chronic fatigue. Crowded minds, like crowded schedules, must be put in orderly array.

One piece of excess mental baggage we can all do without is the unpleasant past. The continual recounting of past failures and shortcomings, like an albatross about the neck, has throttled the potential of many a promising person. It is mandatory that past experiences (including failures, from which we also learn) be accepted as stepping stones to better things, a part of the sail of life rather than an anchor. The mind constantly befogged with self-recrimination about what might have been is a tired mind, operating at minimal efficiency. The least one can do for his mental prowess, paraphrasing the far more noble purpose of Paul the Apostle, is to "forget those things which are past and press forward" toward a mark. The inability to do so is a serious deterrent to coping with chronic fatigue, and may require professional attention.

Improve Ability to Cope

I have a young son who developed an avid interest in tennis at age ten. From the time he first lost a set to me, he was filled with a sense of frustration from which no amount of lecturing would rid him. He vowed to beat me some day, and after several years of intense effort and work, beat me he did, and beat me he now does with ease. Similarly the individual who finds his job stressful because it is beyond the scope of his training may, by intense effort and further training, eventually be able to beat the job. You should, of course, be certain that the goal you set is realistic and attainable, and that it is pursued along fruitful lines. For example, if Dr. Isabel, a family doctor, suddenly decides to become a brain surgeon, she must do so along prescribed channels; working on dogs in the garage is a waste of time.

The incompletely trained person should realize, before he ever gets into a chosen field, that he is at a handicap. The surgeon, for example, who attempts to do surgery without full and total training, is in for a long fight with a short stick. Though additional time and effort and expense may seem to be the more difficult route to go when you are in a period of preparation, it should be realized that, in today's society, anything less than full equipment is a background for stress. It is comparable to sending a soldier to battle without all his gear. Sooner or later, if he fights long enough, he will need what he has not been given, but in the heat of battle there is no time to look around for it. The maxim, then, is this: however costly it may seem at the time, equip yourself as completely as possible for the task you have chosen before you enter the fray! More often than not, the person who interrupts training to go to work, with the intent of finishing up later, never gets back at all. Full and complete training not only means less stress and tension along the way, but it more than pays for itself in the long run.

Of course you should never consider your training complete, in the sense of discontinuing all efforts at bettering the mind or abilities or skills. You should always be the student. The library, educational TV, radio, tapes, seminars, correspondence courses, night school—whatever—all provide a means for the individual to improve his ability to cope and thus reduce stress and tension.

Emotional tension is naturally decreased as one's ability to cope is increased. Frustrations, hostilities, and anxieties are the inevitable by-products of inability to wrestle on even terms with the task at hand. John was a realtor who had a very poor grasp of contracts. He had fouled up one or two deals so badly that he was now quite unsure of himself. He took it upon himself to attend a night class in contract law at the law school in a nearby city, and although he did not comprehend all the legal technicalities involved, he came away with more than enough understanding of contracts to make him feel at ease in a real estate transaction. The tension that had surrounded him in drawing up a deal prior to his training now disappeared, and in its place was self-assurance and confidence.

There is little reason for you to continue in anxiety about doing your chosen work. Communication, teaching material, and learning facilities are so highly developed and widespread that the primary limiting factor is your own desire.

The same is true of fields other than work. Family relationships, peer relationships, even recreational rewards, can all be improved by means available to all if the will is there. The library, the TV, radio, school, the trained professional, and helpful organizations are within reach of everyone. If a given tension-fatigue situation can be remedied by improving your ability to cope, there is little room for sympathizing if you refuse to utilize the means so readily available to any and all who are willing to take the first step.

Provide Tension Outlets

In spite of your best efforts to prevent the mounting of tension, tension is an inevitable part of living, and you must therefore have ready means for its release. Failure to so provide is comparable to building a boiler without a safety valve. Release of tension may proceed along physical, mental, or emotional lines.

Physical Exercise

It can be said without fear of contradiction that physical exercise of proper intensity and duration is the best means of combatting tension available to man. A review of Figure 5 on page 43 shows why this is true. The buildup of tension, with its resultant higher levels of blood pressure, pulse, and muscle tension (see Figure 9), is a common by-product of the vicious cycle in which the Sams of modern civilization find themselves day after day, month after month, year after year. The physiologic purpose of tension is, as you have seen, to adapt the organism for fight or flight. And exercise is commonly the only socially acceptable form of fight-or-flight response available to the Sams of our highly industrialized nations. It alone affords a ready means of utilization of the the stored-up pressure and release of pent-up tensions for the purpose for which they were originally designed—vigorous muscular action. Under its physiologic influence blood pressures trend downward, resting pulse rates decline, muscle tensions vanish, anxieties tend to disappear, and with the restful relaxation that ensues in the wake of regularly "sweating sinew," tension-fatigue becomes less and less a problem. Any individual with a chronic tension-fatigue problem who fails to utilize a well-tailored physical exercise program as a modality for combatting fatigue, when physically able to do so (and 95 percent of persons are), is depriving himself of an irreplaceable tool in his fight against fatigue. For it there is simply no substitute.

Many excellent books are available to the layman in search of a good physical fitness program. Become familiar with one or more of them and put their preachments into effect.

1. Kenneth H. Cooper, M.D., *The New Aerobics*
   Bantam Books, Inc.
   666 Fifth Avenue
   New York, New York 10019

2. Mildred and Kenneth H. Cooper, M.D., *Aerobics for Women*
   (see first reference)

3. M.F. Graham, M.D., *Prescription for Life*
   David McKay Co., Inc.
   750 Third Avenue
   New York, New York 10017

4. Wm. J. Bowerman and W.E. Harris, M.D., *Jogging*
   Grosset and Dunlap, Inc.
   51 Madison Avenue
   New York, New York 10010

5. F.R. Roby and R.P. Davis, *Jogging for Fitness and Weight Control*
   W.B. Saunders Co.
   West Washington Square
   Philadelphia, Pennsylvania 19105

6. Peter Elson, BPE, *Chatelaine's Fitness Plan for Women*
   481 University Avenue
   Toronto, M5W 1A7 Canada

7. *Adult Physical Fitness*
   President's Council on Physical Fitness
   US Government Printing Office
   Washington, D.C. 20402

8. William Hillcourt, *Your Guide to Fitness*
   Golden Press
   Western Publishing Company
   850 Third Avenue
   New York, New York 10022

9. Howard Knuttgen, PhD and David Shepro, PhD, *Complete Conditioning: The No-Nonsense Guide to Fitness and Good Health*
   Addison-Wesley Publishing Co., Inc.
   Reading, Massachusetts 01867

10. Lois Ellfeldt, PhD and Charles LeRoy Lowman, M.D., FACS, *Exercises for the Mature Adult*
    Charles C. Thomas
    301-27 E. Lawrence Avenue
    Springfield, Illinois 62717

There are certain general principles covered in these books which it is well to briefly state here, principles which recount what the listed references explain in detail.

1. There is a level of exercise, in terms of intensity and duration, which is right for you. Failing to reach and maintain this level on a regular basis leaves you short of the optimum exercise effect. Exceeding it, on the other hand, can impose undue physical fatigue.

2. This level, for any given individual, should be reached through a process of conditioning, which must be more gradual (achieved over a longer period of time) in the older or physically impaired person.

3. Before beginning any physical fitness program, it is essential that a careful physical examination precede. If you are over thirty-five and unaccustomed to vigorous exercise, stress testing is desirable to determine the level of activity best suited for you.

4. An effective exercise program should be built around aerobic types of exercise in which the heart and lungs are pushed to a level of activity, in terms of both intensity and duration, compatible with your age and physiologic capacity. Such exercises practically always involve the large leg muscles, as in walking, jogging, running, swimming, tennis, skiing, and the like.

5. Once you have become conditioned to your level of activity, it must become a part of your routine in life, day in, day out; week in, week out; month in, month out; year in, year out. It must become so much a part of your way of life that it is as routine as brushing your teeth.

6. It is essential that the activity be engaged in at least every other day, if not every day, inasmuch as the effects of exercise cannot be stored in a physiologic bank. This activity should ideally increase your pulse rate to about 60 to 80 percent of the pulse range for your age* for at least several minutes.

7. The activity or activities chosen must be flexible and adaptible to different seasons of the year, times of the day, and your schedule.

Persons who have successfully instituted a physical fitness program as a regular part of their daily routine are eventually able to use it in much the same manner that the pill-hound swallows a tranquilizer. You are able to discern when your fatigue is chiefly physical or chiefly emotional (tension), and use exercise accordingly as a ready means of relaxation and release from tension. A doctor, after being awakened at night by a patient, would find it difficult to return to sleep. The next day, he would feel exceedingly weary, out of all proportion to the amount of sleep actually lost. He became engaged in a physical fitness program and eventually made the startling discovery that the fatigue he felt following such nights (when he was awakened) could be wonderfully relieved by a twenty-minute run. Originally he had ascribed his fatigue to lack of sleep. While sleep may have been a factor, tension in the form of a subconscious concern about the patient was far more of one.

Norma was somewhat of a hypochondriacal individual who was constantly beset with vague aches and pains. She slept poorly, was always tired, and was in one or another doctor's office almost constantly. She took up tennis, albeit reluctantly, at the insistence of a neighbor, and as her game improved, so did her disposition. Her visits to the doctor, like her aches and pains, became less and less frequent, and her fatigue disappeared as her sleeping pills went down the disposal. True stories of this type are commonplace in the annals of persons familiar with the fitness field. Your doctor owes it to you to recommend carefully prescribed programs of physical activity, and the individual suffering from chronic fatigue will have fallen far short of the mark if he attempts to deal with his fatigue problem without benefit of vigorous physical activity—as vigorous, that is, as age and conditioning permit.

The helpless, passive feeling so common to depressions result from unpleasant, painful, frustrating life experiences over which you have no control. Even in these instances, people have found physical exercise to be of inestimable value in offsetting the fatigue and the inactivity that results, and in helping themselves to develop a more virile, aggressive attitude toward their problems. The depressed person, the person whose job is filled with frustra-

*Pulse range = maximum heart rate for age minus resting heart rate. (Maximum heart rates for age can be determined from the accompanying table.) Example: Joe has a resting pulse rate (RPR) of 60, a maximal heart rate of 180. His pulse range (PR) is therefore 120 (180−60). 60 percent of the PR (120) = 72. 60 (RPR) + 72 = 132. This is the target pulse rate which Joe should achieve during exercise.

MAXIMUM ATTAINABLE HEART RATE ACCORDING TO AGE

Mean Age	Mean Maximum Heart Rate
20	190
25	185
35	180
45	175
55	170
65	160

The maximum attainable heart rate in man declines gradually with age. For any given individual at a given age, the maximum rate may be as much as 10 to 20 above or below the mean rate.

tions, does much better to take his problems to the tennis court or the jogging track than to attempt to drown them in a cocktail glass. The individual whose chief problem is getting out of bed in the morning due to lack of motivation or challenge might far better start the day with a good swim or run than a heavy breakfast and a pot of coffee and a pep pill. Fatigue founded in the emotions has as its handmaidens inactivity, passivity, helplessness, and despair. In vigorous muscular action you can find the counterparts to all such emotions—action, activity, ability to move, and ability to achieve. Muscles in motion prove to a person, it seems, that the ability to move, to accept challenge, to perform under stress, are not lost, and frequently provide the initiative for action that spreads into other walks of life.

A psychiatrist who was an avid jogger once said about running, "There's been many a day when the only difference in my being in the psychiatrist's chair or on the couch has been a pound of sweat." Years later I developed a health problem that led to despairing moments, and it was only after I, too, became a runner that I fully understood what he meant. Truly the tensions and anxieties and frustrations that so easily beset us do tend to melt away in the fires of vigorous muscular activity. Indeed "honest sweat cleanseth more than the skin; it cleanseth the mind and soul as well."

By chase our long-lived fathers earned their food;
Toil strung the nerves and purified the blood.
But we, their sons, a pampered race of men,
Are dwindled down to three score years and ten.
Better to hunt in fields for health unbought
Than fee the doctor for a nauseous draught.
The wise for cure on exercise depend;
God never made his work for man to mend.

John Dryden (about 1700)

Mental Outlets

Diversions of a mental type have already been mentioned in Chapter 11. The pursuit of other lines of endeavor than those which form your chief occupation or profession is an excellent means of reducing tension via mental outlets. The mind is like a muscle in that it must be exercised to the fullest to keep it in shape, and with mental exercise, as with physical, comes release of tension. Whether mental pursuits outside of your line of work form a diversion, an avocation, or a second mode of income, the end effect is the same. It is impossible for anxiety and tension to occupy the same room of your mind as serious, constructive thought.

Plunging into mental endeavor does not mean settling down before a TV to celebrate at the level of a grade-schooler for hours on end. Absorbing and acceptable and relaxing as such activity is for reasonable periods of time, megadoses of such mind-idling, so characteristic of our affluent society, do not solve the chronic fatigue problem, for mentally and physically, at least, you are no farther along when you finish such a session than when you began. The mind remains unchallenged, problems unsolved. In mental action, as in physical, you convert passivity into activity; mental gymnastics promote mental fertility, and mental fertility engenders creativity; and in creativity there is release from everyday pressures and frustrations. The active mind, as the active body, discovers with each new venture that it can challenge and conquer. So long as you can explore new worlds with your mind, stagnation and despair can never take total charge.

Consider the case of Jesse, a physician in general practice who found the day-in, day-out routine of sore throats and coughs and aches and pains rather tedious. Jesse had always liked mathematics, but never had the opportunity to study calculus in school. So he signed up for a correspondence course in calculus and spent his spare evenings learning the ins and outs of integration and differentiation. Therein he found complete release of tensions that built up during the day.

Tina was a housewife who lost her husband from a heart attack at a fairly young age. Despondency and would-be depression reared their ugly heads. She signed up for some courses at a local university, and in the challenge of learning found eventual release from the tensions that crowded down upon her.

Lucy was a neurosurgeon who, in her sixties, found the schedule she had been keeping too pressure-packed for her years. So she took up writing and in the course of a few years had a brand new career which enabled her to get "out from under" much of her surgical load.

Yes, the mind must be challenged, stimulated, on a regular and organized basis, else it, like splinted muscles, will atrophy and wither and die.

TM, Relaxation Response, Yoga, and Self-Hypnosis

Recent years have seen a renewal of interest in modes of freeing the mind from the entanglements of time and place. Some of these techniques, such as TM and the RR,* employ a key sound, a symbol, or word repetition in a quiet environment with the person at complete rest to promote complete release, or rather deconcentration, of the mind—a dissociation from the pressurized environment through association with transcendent thoughts and ideas. Such techniques are not new. They are found in many of the Far Eastern cultures, dating back centuries. Basically they are a form of self-hypnosis, and as in hypnosis, the parameters of tension—blood pressure, pulse rate, and muscle tension—all fall to resting levels. There is good scientific evidence that many of these techniques, properly employed, have a pronounced tension-releasing effect.

The technique for muscle relaxation for induction of sleep described in Chapter 6 may be utilized as a means of begetting mental tranquility if you sit or kneel or squat in a comfortable position instead of lying down, since recumbency invites sleep. Whatever the posture assumed, you should allow for comfort for a minimum of twenty or thirty minutes. Other key requisites for relaxation, as pointed out by Dr. Benson** of Harvard University, are absolute quiet, some object (such as a key word or a symbol) on which thought can be concentrated to the exclusion of all other thought processes, and an attitude of total passivity. The passive attitude, says Dr. Benson, is most important of all.

That such books as those dealing with transcendental meditation and the relaxation response have made best-seller lists for months is mute evidence of the endless search of mankind for release from tension. You could do worse than familiarize yourself with such works, being careful to keep them in proper perspective.

Emotional Outlets

Certain types of physical activity serve as a release for emotionally produced tension, either as a participant or spectator. The tennis player, for example, has been likened by some psychiatrists to a combatant who bludgeons his opponent at long range with the tennis racquet as his weapon.

*TM: transcendental meditation. RR: relaxation response.

**Herbert Benson, MD, *The Relaxation Response* (New York: Morrow, 1975).

The winning placement, the disarming serve, the powerful overhead are not only blows that win the point, but outlets that release pent-up aggressions and hostilities, dating back to when man used a leopard femur to subdue his enemies. The football player, slamming into his opposition with all the fierceness of an iron-clad gladiator of old, is aggression personified. In the bone-crushing tackle, the bruising block, or the skillful interception of a pass, he downs an enemy or denies him his goal, and finds in his art sweet release. The runner, in contrast to the tennis player or footballer who stands and fights, flees from his tensions. He outruns them, as it were, but finds in so doing the same release from tension as the vis-a-vis combatant.

The spectator at a football, basketball, or other game in which a favorite player or team is participating, finds much of the same release (though far from the same degree as the participant) as is found by the player(s) or team with which he identifies. Joe may be too old, too obese, and too out of shape to slam his body at the opposition, but in identifying with a team or player, he participates vicariously in the sport. Emotionally, at least, he flings himself at the opposition with the same wild abandon as the player, exults in the same sweet release of victory, and pouts in the same bitter dregs of defeat. Thus spectating has its emotional benefits, but it falls far short of active participation in vigorous muscular endeavor.

In this regard motion pictures, TV, and radio can afford emotional release. One physician spends his off afternoons in a movie theater, completely engrossed in the goings-on on the screen. He finds a complete emotional release from the tensions of life. But here, again, in such passivity there is danger when carried to extremes. Identification measures, vicarious pursuits, and imaginary encounters, while they have their place when used wisely, cannot replace active pursuits with the body, the intellect, or the emotions. For example, hours upon hours of TV watching, while providing some emotional release, carry with them a dangerous inertia which, in the long run, can but lead to deterioration of the spectator. All such outlets should be meted out judiciously, with much the same expertise that a good cook allots ingredients to a cake.

The development of artistic or creative instincts can do much to provide release from emotional tensions. One physician found his channel of release in a home electric organ, the playing of which he took up at the ripe age of sixty-five. Many are those who have taken up the artist's brush and seen their tensions fade into the paint splayed upon the canvas. Paralleling such active participation is acquaintance with the great artists and great art, great musicians and great music—in other words art and music appreciation.

In the world of literature you can find both mental and emotional release. Good books are economical, easily available doorways into other worlds—worlds of amazement and wonder, both fictional and real. They can be stepping stones to new achievements, a ladder to new understandings, windows to the mind and soul. To neglect such a ready outlet of tension is comparable to looking for your glasses when they reside on the end of your nose. The experience(s) of lifetimes are veritably at your fingertips in the libraries.

Improve Philosophy

To a large degree, your philosophy of life determines the manner in which you react to a given stress. The hedonist may try to shrug off problems as but temporary hitches in the search for happiness. The fatalist likewise, in a more somber vein, accepts "whatever will be will be" and trudges along, viewing the ups and downs of life as the way it is. "Do the best you can and that's all you can do" has a lot to be said for it from a materialistic point of view. But when the going gets really rough, no man-made philosophy can offer the ultimate solutions or fulfill all the following criteria to buffer you against the stresses of life:

1. Protect against the detours and exigencies of life.
2. Replace a win-at-all-cost attitude with that of giving your best to the total life situation.
3. Provide a source of strength beyond your human capacity.
4. Recognize the manifold nature and needs of your own self and your fellow beings.
5. Take the long look and put life in its proper perspective.
6. Provide a real reason for being.

Through the ages philosophers have lived and died, their philosophies come and gone, mute testimony to the fallibility of man-made credos and the flimsy nature of human solutions. Human efforts to solve the deepest dilemmas of life have all come up wanting, primarily because they "see through a glass darkly." When the finite mind attempts to attain infinite truth with finite knowledge, the result is fallibility, incompleteness, and, ultimately, despair. Nobel prize-winner Francis Crick had this to say: ". . .to those of you who may be vitalists I would make this prophecy: what everyone believed yesterday and you believe today, only cranks will believe tomorrow." Truth—total truth—is a verity beyond the comprehension and grasp of the human mind. It was a lowly Galilean who said; "I am the way, the truth, and the life!" Could this be an answer to our fretting and fuming, to our anxieties, our stress—our chronic fatigue? "Come unto me, all ye that labor and are heavy-laden—and I will give you rest."

Postlude

Chronic fatigue—that nagging, worn-out feeling that hangs like an albatross about the necks of millions of Americans day after day after day—is a subjective feeling which may result from organic, physiologic, mental, or emotional causes, or any combination of these. By far the majority of cases stem from emotional sources, born of a complex interaction of you with your environment as you press toward a goal or goals. The result of such interaction is stress, which in turn begets anxiety, which gives birth to fatigue (the tension-fatigue syndrome). The underlying physiologic mechanism is that of the fight-or-flight response to threatening stimuli, a response which is acted out again and again in your effort to adapt to a constantly changing situation as you pursue your goal.

Repetition of acute stressful stimuli leads, over a period of years, to a state of exhaustion or near-exhaustion. It is this state in which too many inhabitants of industrialized (civilized) societies such as our own find themselves today. When man's goals were simple—pursuit of a quarry with a club—the release of tension was quick and sure. But with the advance of civilization goals have become complex and elusive, and the resultant chronic stress manifests itself as chronic tension, whether in society as a whole or in its individual members. It is axiomatic that chronic tension produces chronic fatigue, and that relief of fatigue can come only with release of tension. It is to this end—the release of tension—that measures for relief of fatigue must be directed. Such release must follow along many avenues in societies where people, their environments, and their goals are as complex as in our own.

In the process of becoming involved in complex goal situations, sound principles of good health—rest, nutrition, and recreation—are commonly abandoned or neglected. The successful combatting of chronic fatigue requires that such principles be put into operation again. Although complete abolition of chronic fatigue is seldom possible unless radical measures are taken, much relief can be obtained.

It is with these basic tenets—intelligent understanding of the problem and logical measures for relief—that this book has concerned itself. Assiduous application of its contents cannot help but bring some measure of relief from this bane of modern existence—chronic fatigue.

Appendices

APPENDIX 1

Desirable Weight According to Height

DESIRABLE WEIGHT ACCORDING TO HEIGHT (Age 25 and over)*

Height	Weight in Pounds (in Indoor Clothing)		
	Small Frame	Medium Frame	Large Frame
(1-inch heels)		Men	
5 feet 2 inches	112-220	118-129	126-141
3	115-123	121-133	129-144
4	118-126	124-136	132-148
5	121-129	127-139	135-152
6	124-133	130-143	138-156
7	128-137	134-147	142-161
8	132-141	138-152	147-166
9	136-145	142-156	151-170
10	140-150	146-160	155-174
11	144-154	150-165	159-179
6 feet 0 inches	148-158	154-170	164-184
1	152-162	158-175	168-189
2	156-167	162-180	173-194
3	160-171	167-185	178-199
4	164-175	172-190	182-204

* "New Weight Standards for Men and Women," Metropolitan Life Insurance Co., Statistical Bulletin, Nov.-Dec. 1959. Reprinted with permission.

DESIRABLE WEIGHT ACCORDING TO HEIGHT (Age 25 and over)

(2-inch heels)		Women	
4 feet 10 inches	92-98	96-107	104-119
11	94-101	98-110	106-122
5 feet 0 inches	96-104	101-113	109-125
1	99-107	104-116	112-128
2	102-110	107-119	115-131
3	105-113	110-122	118-134
4	108-116	113-126	121-138
5	111-119	116-130	125-142
6	114-123	120-135	129-146
7	118-127	124-139	133-150
8	122-131	128-143	137-154
9	126-135	132-147	141-158
10	130-140	136-151	145-163
11	134-144	140-155	149-168
6 feet 0 inches	138-148	144-159	153-173

APPENDIX 2

Energy-Cost of Activity

ENERGY-COST OF ACTIVITY (in Calories)* **

Intensity of Exercise	Hour
Low	70-150
Sleeping	70
Sitting	100
Standing	110
Sitting (handwork)	120
Driving a car (pleasure)	140
Mild	150-300
Pool	162
Horseback riding	170
Walking 2 mph	192
House painting	210
Gardening	220
Carpentry	230
Canoeing	230
Horseshoes	240
Bicycling 5½ mph	240
Dancing (modern)	250
Golf	250
Lawn mowing (power)	250
Domestic work	250
Walking 2½ mph	256
Mowing (hand)	270
Moderate	300-499
Rowing 2½ mph (pleasure)	300
Fencing	300
Hiking 2½ mph – 20 pounds	300
Walking 3 mph	300
Swimming crawl 20 yards/minute	300
Breast 20 yards/minute	300
Back 25 yards/minute	300

*Based on average man 5 feet 8 inches tall, weight 150-160 pounds.

**From Charles T. Kuntzleman, *Activetics*, (New York: Peter Wyden, 1975). Reprinted with permission.

Intensity of Exercise	Hour
Moderate (continued)	
Archery	312
Hiking 3 mph – 20 pounds	312
Walking 3½ mph	315
Weeding	336
Hiking 3 mph – 40 pounds	348
Walking 4 mph	348
Badminton (recreational)	350
Volleyball (recreational)	350
Skating, ice and roller (leisure)	350
Table tennis	360
Hiking 3½ mph – 20 pounds	380
Baseball pitching	390
Pick and shovel	400
Horseback riding (trot)	415
Canoeing 4 mph	420
Square dancing	420
Swimming crawl 30 yards/minute	420
Tennis (recreational)	426
Moderate High	450-599
Swimming breast 30 yards/minute	450
Back 30 yards/minute	450
Walking 4½ mph	450
Sawing	480
Water skiing	480
Digging and shoveling	500
Polka dancing	540
Swimming back 35 yards/minute	540
Side 30 yards/minute	550
Skiing (downhill)	594
High	600-749
Badminton (competitive)	600
Handball	600
Swimming breast 40 yards/minute	600
Mountain climbing	600
Soccer	600
Tennis (competitive)	600
Volleyball (competitive)	600
Basketball	608

Intensity of Exercise	Hour
Football (playground)	611
Squash	612
Fencing	630
Skating (vigorously)	640
Bicycling 13 mph	660
Running 5.5 mph (jogging)	660
Swimming side 40 yards/minute	660
Back 40 yards/minute	660
Swimming crawl 45 yards/minute	660
Running 7.2 mph	720
Skiing on level 5 mph	720
Very High	750+
Wrestling and combatives	790
Running 8 mph	825
Swimming crawl 55 yards/minute	840
Sculling (racing)	840
Running 8.7 mph	900
Rowboating (racing)	970
Rowing machine (very vigorous)	972
Running in place 140 counts/minute	1500
Swimming crawl 65 yards/minute	1600
Running in place 160 counts/minute	1800

APPENDIX 3

The Basic Four Food Groups

THE BASIC FOUR FOOD GROUPS*

A Daily Guide

No single food contains all the substances necessary for the normal growth of children. Therefore, choosing wisely for children's diets means selecting foods from all four of the basic four food groups.

Why are foods divided into groups? Because these groups point out the main kinds of foods to include in our meals each day.

How are foods divided into groups? Generally on the basis of their major nutritional contributions to the diet.

THE MEAT GROUP

Meats offer protein, the B vitamins, and iron. These essentials are needed for growing tall, for building muscles, for important body functions, and for the formation of hemoglobin in the red blood cells. Chicken, fish, eggs, and peanut butter can be used instead of meat to provide protein and other important nutrients in the diet. Cheese, like meat, is a good source of protein and, like milk, is also a good source of calcium.

THE MILK GROUP

Milk contains protein, calcium, phosphorus, riboflavin, and vitamin A. In addition, fortified milk contains vitamin D. These nutrients promote growth, build strong bones and teeth, provide energy, and help maintain smooth, healthy skin and good eyesight.

THE BREAD AND CEREAL GROUP

Bread and cereals are good sources of energy for the endless activity of children. They also contain protein. Whole grain or restored bread and cereals are valuable sources of iron and B vitamins. Enriched cornmeal and converted rice also contain B vitamins and iron. Servings of breads, cereals, noodles, and other foods in this group easily fit into many meal patterns and become very satisfying and appealing complements to other foods.

*From *Meal Planning for Young Children,* Nutritional Service, General Mills, Inc., Minneapolis, Minnesota.

THE VEGETABLE AND FRUIT GROUP

Vegetables and fruits have a variety of virtues. They furnish a substantial share of the vitamins and they are valuable as roughage. Vitamin C helps build and maintain healthy gums, body tissues, and blood vessels, helps resist infection, and aids in healing. Vitamin A is important for normal vision and to keep skin and mucous membranes healthy.

THE EXTRA FOOD GROUP

Some familiar foods not included in the groups are by custom a part of meals. For example, fats and sugars are useful in cooking and flavoring. They provide energy (calories) and add variety. With the exception of butter, which contains vitamin A, fats and sugars are poor sources of vitamins and minerals, and they contain no protein.

FOUR BASIC FOOD GROUPS FOR PLANNING OF DAILY DIET

Proper nutrition begins with meeting daily requirements from the following four food groups. Wise meal planning should always start here.

Food Group	Best Food Sources	Substitutes or Equivalents	Daily Requirements
Milk	Milk and milk products (cheese, buttermilk, ice cream)	8 oz. glass of milk. 1½ ozs. cheese or 1½ cups cottage cheese	Children under 9: 2 to 3 cups Children 9-12: 3 or more cups Teenagers: 4 or more cups Adults: 2 or more cups Pregnant women: 3 or more cups Lactating women: 4 or more cups Elderly: 1 cup
Meat	Beef, veal, lamb, pork, fish, fowl, shellfish, liver	Milk, eggs, most cheese, dry beans, dry peas, nuts 1 oz. meat = 1 egg or 1 oz. cheese or 8 ozs. milk	2 or more servings (4 to 8 ozs.) per day Child: 2 servings Teenager: 4 or more servings Adult: 1 to 2 servings Elderly: 1 serving

Meat (continued)			1 serving = 2 to 3 ozs. lean cooked meat, poultry, or fish; 2 eggs; 1 cup cooked dried beans; 4 tablespoons peanut butter
Vegetables and Fruits	All vegetables and fruits	Citrus fruits: 4 ozs. orange juice = 1 orange = ½ grapefruit = 8 ozs. tomato juice = 4 ozs. grapefruit juice	1 serving (4 oz.) citrus fruits and 2 other fruits Child: 1 serving Teenager: 2 servings Adult: 1 serving Elderly: 1 or more servings
		Other fruits: 1 serving = 1 apple, pear, banana, peach, or nectarine = ¼ cantaloupe = 2 plums = 15 large cherries = 10 large strawberries = 1 bunch grapes	
	Green leafy-yellow vegetable: 1 serving = ½ to 2/3 cup asparagus, broccoli, brussel sprouts, butternut squash, carrots, chicory, endive, escarole, hubbard squash, parsley, peppers, pumpkin, watercress, beet greens, collard, dandelion, kale, lettuce, mustard greens, sweet potatoes		One serving of a green leafy-yellow vegetable and One serving of an "other vegetable" -or- Two servings of green leafy-yellow vegetable
	"Other" vegetable: 1 serving = ½ cup beets, cabbage, cauliflower, celery, cucumber, eggplant, lettuce, onions, peas, radishes, rutabaga, sauerkraut, strong beans, tomatoes, turnip (yellow)		For everyone

FOUR BASIC FOOD GROUPS FOR PLANNING OF DAILY DIET

Breads and Cereals	Breads, cooked cereals, packaged cereals, cornmeal, crackers, flour, grits, macaroni, spaghetti, noodles, rice, rolled oats, foods baked with whole grain or enriched flour	1 serving = 1 slice enriched bread = 1 muffin (2 inches diam.) = 2 graham crackers = 5 saltine crackers = 6 melba toast rounds = 1 baked potato of 2 inches diam. = ½ cup mashed potato = ¼ cup baked beans = 1/3 cup corn = ¾ cup dry cereal = ½ cup cooked cereal = ½ to 3/4 cup noodles, rice, etc.	Two to four servings (adjusted to caloric needs) Child: 4 servings Teenager: more than 4 servings Adult: 4 servings Elderly: 2 servings

OTHER FOODS (To Be Used Sparingly)

Fats	Margarine, butter, dressings, oils, shortenings. (The child should have 2 tablespoons of, preferably, margarine per day, the teenager 4 tablespoons, the adult 2, the elderly 1.)
Desserts	Cookies made with molasses, oatmeal or raisins, gingerbread, puddings, fruit cups, custards, and Jell-o (an excellent source of protein).
Sugars	Candy, soft drinks, fruit-flavored beverages, honey, jam, jelly, frostings, icings.

APPENDIX 4

Basic Meal Pattern

BASIC MEAL PATTERN*

Breakfast	Fruit or juice Meat or substitute Bread or cereal Margarine Milk
Lunch	Salad Meat or substitute Vegetable Margarine Dessert (include fruit) Milk
Dinner	Salad Meat or substitute Vegetable Bread or substitute Margarine Fruit or equivalent dessert Milk

*Ibid.

Bibliography

Adamson, G. L. "Fatigue." *Journal of Aviation Medicine* 23 (1952): 584-88.

"Adipocyte Increase at Critical Time Key to Obesity." *Pediatric News,* June 1975, p. 12.

Agricultural Research Service, U.S. Dept. of Agriculture. *Nutrition – Up to Date, Up to You.* Wash. D.C.: U.S. Gov't. Printing Office.

Alvarez, W. C. "What Is the Matter with the Patient Who Is Chronically Tired?" *J Missouri MA* 38 (1941): 365-68.

Bartley, S. H. "Conflict, Frustration, and Fatigue." *Psychosomatic Medicine* 5 (1943): 160-65.

____. "Fatigue and Inadequacy." *Physiol Rev* 37 (1957): 301-24.

____, and Chute, E. "A Preliminary Classification of the Concept of Fatigue." *Psychol Rev* 52 (1945): 169-74.

Basmajian, J. V. "Biofeedback: The Clinical Tool Behind the Catchword." *Modern Medicine,* 1 October 1976, pp. 61-64.

Benson, H. *The Relaxation Response.* New York: Wm. Morrow & Co., 1975.

Berger, R. A. "Comparison between Two Methods in Recovery from Muscular Fatigue." *J Amer Correction Therapy* 24 (1970): 73.

Best, C. H., and Taylor, N. B. *Physiological Basis of Medical Practice.* Baltimore: Williams & Wilkins Co., 1945.

Brean, Herbert. *How to Stop Smoking.* New York: Pocket Books, 1975.

Bricklin, M. "Vitamin C Keeps Arteries Youthful." *Prevention,* January 1976, pp. 37-44.

Campbell, A.; Converse, P.; and Kahn, R. L., eds. *The Meaning of Work: Interpretation and Proposals for Measurement in the Meaning of Social Change.* New York: Basic Books, Inc., 1972.

Carron, A. V. "Physical Fatigue and Motor Learning." *Research Quarterly* 40 (1969): 682-86.

Cohen, J. "Sleep and Insomnia." *JAMA*, 16 August 1976, pp. 875-76.

Collipp, P. J., ed. "Obesity in Childhood and Adolescence." *Pediatric Annals*, May 1975.

Committee on Nutritional Misinformation, National Academy of Sciences. "Hazards of Overuse of Vitamin D." *Pediatric Currents*, October 1975.

"Compliance and Prescribance." *Am J Dis Child*, September 1975, p. 1009.

Cooper, Kenneth M. *The New Aerobics.* New York: Evans & Co., 1970.

Crosby, Wm. H. "Can a Vegetarian Be Well Nourished?" *JAMA*, 25 August 1975, p. 898.

Cureton, T. K., Jr. *Physical Fitness and Dynamic Health.* New York: Dell Publishing Co., Inc., 1967.

David, H. "Symposium on Fatigue: Introductory Remarks." *Psychosomatic Medicine* 5: 152-54.

Dement, W. C., and Guilleminault, C. "Sleep Disorders: The State of the Art." *Hospital Practice*, November 1973, pp. 57-71.

Dill, D. B. "The Nature of Fatigue." *Geriatrics* 10 (1955): 474-78.

DiPalme, J. R. "Rx: Malnutrition." *Current Prescribing*, August 1977, pp. 54-57.

Economic Research Service. *Home Grown Fruits and Vegetables.* Reprinted from *Vegetable Situation*. Wash. D.C.: U.S. Department of Agriculture, 1976.

Elrick, H., et al. "Indians Who Run 100 Miles on 1500 Calories a Day." *The Physician & Sports Med*, February 1976, pp. 38-42.

Enelow, Allen J., ed. *Depression in Medical Practice.* West Point, Pa.: Merck Sharp & Dohme, 1970.

____, and Wexler, M. *Psychiatry in the Practice of Medicine*. New York: Oxford University Press, 1966.

Ergonomics Research Society. "Symposium on Fatigue." *Lancet* 868 (1952).

Eversharp, Inc. *Alcohol: Who Is Allergic?* Annual Report, revised. Culver City, California: Schick Safety Razor Co., 1966.

"Exercise and Aging." *Phys Fitness Res Digest*, April 1977.

Floyd, W. F., and Welford, A. T., eds. "Psychologic Criteria of Fatigue." *Symposium on Fatigue*. London: H. K. Lewis, 1953.

Forbes, W. H. "Problems Arising in Study of Fatigue." *Psychosomatic Medicine*, April 1943, pp. 155-57.

Fried, John J. *The Vitamin Conspiracy*. New York: E. P. Dutton & Co., Inc., 1975.

Friedlander, H. S. "Fatigue as a Presenting Symptom: Management in General Practice." *Curr Therap Res* 4 (1962): 443-49.

Globus, C. G. "Sleep Duration and Feeling State." *Int Psychiat Clin* 7 (1970): 78-84.

Goodman, L., and Gilman, A. *The Pharmacological Basis of Therapeutics.* New York: MacMillan, 1941.

Goodnight, F. "Vitamin D Excess Seen Adding to Atherosclerosis Risk." *Medical Tribune*, 25 June 1975, p. 21.

Graham, M. F. *Prescription for Life.* New York: David McKay Co., 1966.

Gray, F. D. *Tea Situation: Trends and Prospects.* Economic Research Service of the U.S. Dept. of Agriculture, Food Consumption and Utilization Section.

Gross, I. H., and Bartley, J. "Fatigue in House Care." *Applied Psychology* 35 (1951): 205-7.

Hagerman, F. C. "An Investigation of Accumulative Acute Fatigue in Participants at the 1966 World Modern Pentathlon Championships, Melbourne." *J Sports Med* 8 (1968): 158-70.

Harms, H. E., and Soniat, T. L. "The Meaning of Fatigue." *Medical Clinics of North America* 36 (1952): 311-17.

Hatterer, L. J. "A Psychiatrist Searches for the Roots of Our Addictions." *Modern Medicine*, 15 October 1975, pp. 53-57.

Helmstra, N. W. "The Effects of Stress Fatigue on Performance in a Simulated Driving Situation." *Ergonomics* 13: 209-13.

Herbert, V. "The Megavitamin Therapy Fad." *Consultant,* May 1977, pp. 70-77.

Herzberg, F., et al. *Motivation to Work.* New York: Wiley-Interscience, 1959.

Hicks, J. T. "Treatment of Fatigue in General Practice." *Clinical Medicine* 71 (1964): 85-90.

Horowitz, I.; Fabry, E. M.; and Gerson, C. D. "Bioavailability of Ascorbic Acid in Orange Juice." *JAMA* 14 June 1976, pp. 2624-25.

Hurwitz, W. M. "Misdiagnosis of Nervous Fatigue." *Geriatrics*, February 1970, p. 57.

"Hyperlipidemia: Care in Child May Prevent Adult Atherosclerosis." *Pediatric News*, Vol. 9, No. 6, p. 5.

"Jogging." *Phys Fitness Res Digest*, January 1977.

"Jogging May Keep Depressives off Therapists Couch." *Medical World News*, 20 March 1978, p. 15.

Kahn, R. L., et al. *Organizational Stress: Studies in Role Conflict and Ambiguity*. New York: Wiley-Interscience, 1964.

Kamman, G. R. "Fatigue as a Symptom in Depressed Patients." *Lancet* 65: 238-40.

Margen, S., and Allen, L. H. "What to Look for in the Nutritional Examination." *Consultant*, March 1976, pp. 43-52.

Martin, P. "The Old Men and Women of the Mountains." *Parade*, 4 April 1976, pp. 10-12.

Mason, J. W. "Organization of Psychoendocrine Mechanisms." *Psychosomatic Medicine* 30 (1968): 565.

Mason, Mary Lou. *Personal Communication*. Indianapolis: Eli Lilly & Co.

McLanahan, Sandra. "Yoga Has Much to Offer Medicine." *Amer Med News*, 11 April 1977, p. 7.

Meal Planning for Young Children. General Mills, Inc., 1966.

"The Medical Effects of Coffee." *Medical World News*, 26 January 1976.

Menninger, Karl A. *Man Against Himself.* New York: Harcourt, Brace, Jovanovich, 1938.

Merton, P. A. "Problems of Muscular Fatigue." *Brit Med Bull* 12 (1956): 3.

Michaels, R. R.; Huber, M. J.; and McCann, D. S. "Evaluation of TM as a Method of Reducing Stress." *Science* 192 (1976): 1242-44.

Miller, J. Z., et al. "Therapeutic Effect of Vitamin C." *JAMA*, 17 January 1977, pp. 248-51.

Miller, Wm. F. "Smoking and Health: A Commentary." *Texas Med*, January 1978, pp. 83-88.

Mines, Sam. "A Psychiatrist Searches for the Roots of our Addictions." *Modern Medicine*, 15 October 1975, pp. 53-57.

Muncie, W. "Chronic Fatigue." *Psychosomatic Medicine* 3 (1941): 277-85.

Nussbaum, H. E. "Chronic Fatigue." *J Med Soc New Jersey* 60 (1963): 499-503.

"Nutrition." *MD*, March 1976, pp. 100-11.

Nutrition. Manhasset, New York: Weight Watchers International, Inc.

"Opened Vitamin C Changes into Hazardous Compounds." *Infectious Diseases*, July 1975.

Oswald, Ian. "Aberrant Sleep: Too Much . . . Too Little." *Drug Therapy*, July 1976, pp. 28-37.

Passmore, R., et al. *Handbook on Human Nutritional Requirements.* WHO Monogr Ser 0(61): 1-66, 1974.

Pathak, C. L. "Muscular Work and Fatigue—a Review." *Indian J Physiol Pharmacol* 13 (1969): 87-97.

Pauling, L. "Are Recommended Daily Allowances for Vitamin C Adequate?" *Proc Natl Acad Sci* 71 (1974): 4442-46.

Pauling, L. "Ascorbic Acid & the Common Cold," Part II. *Medical Tribune*, 7 April 1976.

Pauling, L. "The Case for Vitamin C in Maintaining Health and Preventing Disease." *Modern Medicine*, 1 July 1976, pp. 68-72.

Pauling, L. "The Good Drugs Do." *Medical Tribune.*

Paykel, E. S. "Depression." *Current Prescribing*, January 1978, pp. 68-74.

"Physical Fitness Practices and Programs for Elementary and Secondary Schools." *Phys Fitness Res Digest*, 4 October 1976, Series 6.

Physicians Desk Reference. Oradell, New York: Medical Economics Co., 1976.

"Physiological, Psychological Aspects of Sleep." *Modern Medicine*, 26 August 1968, p. 70.

Pollack, Herbert, and Halpern, Seymour. *Therapeutic Nutrition.* Washington, D.C.: National Academy of Sciences — National Research Council, Pub. 234.

Portis, S. A., and Zitman, I. H. "Mechanism of Fatigue in Neuropsychiatric Patients; preliminary report." *JAMA* 121 (1943): 569-73; abstracted Portis, S. A. *Psychosomatic Medicine* 5 (1943): 158-59.

Power, L. "As Physicians, We Are Too Lax on Nutrition." *Med Opinion*, February 1976, pp. 51-53.

Public Health Service. *The Health Consequences of Smoking.* Washington, D.C.: U.S. Government Printing Office, 1967.

Public Health Service. *Smoking and Health.* Washington, D.C.: U.S. Government Printing Office, Pub. No. 1103.

Rathmann, D. M. *Vegetable Oils in Nutrition.* New York: Corn Products Refining Co., 1973.

Rhoads, J. M. "Overwork." *JAMA*, 13 June 1977, pp. 2615-18.

Roche Laboratories. *The Anatomy of Sleep.* Nutley, New Jersey: Hoffman-LaRoche Inc., 1966.

Rumball, W. M., et al. "Analysis of Running and the Prediction of Ultimate Performance." *Nature* 228 (1970): 184-85.

Sachar, E. J. "Endocrine Changes in Stress and Mental Illness." *Hospital Practice*, July 1975, pp. 49-55.

Schildkraut, J. J. "Biogenic Amines and Affective Disorders." *Annual Review of Medicine* 25 (1974): 333.

Schwab, R. S., and Thomas, D. "Psychiatric Findings in Fatigue." *Am J Psychiatry* 109 (1953): 621-25.

Seligman, M. *Helplessness: On Depression, Development and Death.* San Francisco: W. H. Freeman & Co., 1975.

Selye, Hans. "The Evolution of the Stress Concept." *J Intl Acad Prev Med* 2 (1975): 1.

Selye, Hans, and Stone, H. *On the Experimental Morphology of the Adrenal Cortex.* Springfield: Chas. C. Thomas, 1950.

Selye, Hans. *Stress of Life,* rev. ed. New York: McGraw-Hill, 1976.

Shaw, D. L., Chesney, M. S., et al. "Management of Fatigue: A Physiologic Approach." *Amer J Med Sci* 243 (1962): 758-69.

Sheehan, G. "The Common Roots of Saints and Athletes." *The Physician and Sports Medicine*, February 1978.

Shephard, R. J., and Kavanagh, T. "The Effects of Training on the Aging Process." *The Physician and Sports Medicine*, January 1978.

Shephard, R. J. *Endurance Fitness*, second ed. Toronto, Canada: University of Toronto Press, 1977.

"Smoke Signals." *MD*, October 1975, pp. 51-53.

Smoking and Heart Disease. New York: American Heart Ass'n.

Snook, S. H., et al. "Psychophysiologic Studies of Human Fatigue Criteria." *Human Factors* 11 (1969): 291-300.

Snow, E. W.; Machlow, L. O.; et al. "The Tired Patient." *Medical Times*, November 1959.

"Somnology: A New Clinical Specialty." *MD*, February 1976, pp. 55-61.

Stamler, J. "Primary Prevention of the Major Heart Diseases." *Bulletin of the International Society of Cardiology*, Summer 1975, p. 5.

Steinbaugh, M., and Strong, W. B. "Primary Prevention of Atherosclerosis: Nutritional Aspects." *Southern Medical Journal*, March 1975, p. 328.

Stone, R. A., and DeLeo, J. "Psychotherapeutic Control of Hypertension." *New England Journal of Medicine* 294 (1976): 80-84.

"Stress-Triggered Organic Disease in this Year of Economic Anxiety." *Medical World News*, 24 March 1975.

"The Subtle Killer, Fatigue." *Medical Science Law* 9 (1969): 1-2.

Sullivan, M. W. *From Tension to Relaxation*. Menlo Park, California: Granger-Doyle.

"Swimming and Bicycling." *Phys Fitness Res Digest*.

Tainter, M. L., and Ferris, A. J. *Aspirin in Modern Therapy.* New York: Bayer Co. Division of Sterling Drug, Inc., 1969.

Tappel, A. L. "Vitamin E." *Nutrition Today*, July/August 1973, pp. 4-12.

Winick, M., and Levitas, I. M. "Fighting the Fads, if a Patient Asks about Diet." *Current Prescribing*, December 1977, pp. 68-70.

Tracy, F. E. "The Cyclic Psychosomatic Fatigue Syndrome." *Connecticut Medicine* 24 (1960): 357-59.

"Treating Common Sleep Disorders." *Medical World News*, 5 April 1976, pp. 29-44.

University of South Florida College of Medicine. *Report of Second Wyeth Nutrition Symposium.* Philadelphia: Wyeth Laboratories, 1976.

"Vitamin E Fails in Heart Study." *Medical World News*, 2 May 1977, p. 22.

Welford, A. T. "Psychologic and Physiologic Aspects of Fatigue." *Nature* 169 (1952): 728-29.

Williams, M. H. "Effect of Selected Doses of Alcohol on Fatigue." *Research Quarterly* 40 (1969): 832-40.

Taylor, B. B. "The Fatigued Worker." *Western Medicine* 2 (1961): 535-38.

Wooster, H. A., and Blanck, F. C. *Nutritional Data.* Pittsburgh: H. J. Heinz Co., 1950.

Work in America: A Report of a Special Task Force to the Secretary of Health, Education, and Welfare. Cambridge, Mass.: MIT Press, 1973.

World Demand Prospects for Coffee in 1980. Washington, D.C.: U.S. Department of Agriculture, Foreign Agricultural Report No. 86.

Index